"In her new book, *30 Days of Hope for Joy through a Child's Severe Illness,* author Gale Alexander shares real-life stories that encourage and instill hope. Readers have a front-row seat to witness God's amazing activity in the lives of Gale's granddaughter and five other children who all experience victory in the midst of adversity. These young lives, all living examples of God's miraculous power and tender care, inspire readers to place their hope securely in our great God."

—*Kathy Howard, speaker and author of* Unshakeable Faith *and* Before His Throne

"*30 Days of Hope for Joy through a Child's Severe Illness* is a heart-wrenching and inspiring look at situations that would challenge any believer's faith. Uniquely gifted, Gale Alexander weaves words together in a beautiful pattern to express the conflict of emotions that families can experience when raising a child with special health care needs. In spite of the disappointment and heartache, joy and hope shine through every page. I wish I had the opportunity to read this book when we were raising our child with special needs."

—*Peggy Nikkel, executive director's wife, Wyoming Southern Baptist Convention*

"Gale's book is divine and gives major, positive input to understanding the difficulties and the joy of a family with EB. It is a testament to Ella and the life God has planned for her. It is delightfully written and filled with enchanting stories of courage."

—*Margo Bean, children's book author*

"Gale Alexander's poignant writings about children with severe illnesses melt the heart! Each true story provides the portrait of a child facing his or her individual challenge with youthful courage and optimism. Artful Haiku poetry delicately created by the author highlights the suffering and hope woven into each child's experience. Gale Alexander's faith in God inspires the reader to grow in his or her own faith. The Bible passages she includes illuminate the essence of each story. The account of each child's illness proves that joy can result even from the most heartbreaking of circumstances!"

—*Margaret Benson, The Wyoming Communication Group*

"I haven't been given the accountability of parenting or grandparenting a child with severe illness, but *30 Days of Hope for Joy through a Child's Severe Illness* brought laughter and tears, sorrow and joy, and a deeper appreciation for parents and grandparents whose love enables them to do whatever it takes for their child to experience life to the fullest.
No doubt Gale's grace-filled stories will encourage every parent, grandparent, and friend of an ill child to believe and act on the fact that God can be trusted. God reveals Himself to us in amazing ways, even when He chooses not to heal."

—*Andrea Mullins, former publisher of New Hope® Publishers*

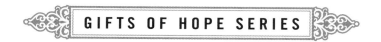

GIFTS OF HOPE SERIES

30 DAYS OF HOPE

FOR JOY THROUGH A CHILD'S SEVERE ILLNESS

GALE ALEXANDER

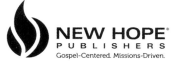

NEW HOPE®
PUBLISHERS
Gospel-Centered. Missions-Driven.

BIRMINGHAM, ALABAMA

New Hope® Publishers
PO Box 12065
Birmingham, AL 35202-2065
NewHopePublishers.com
New Hope Publishers is a division of WMU®.

Library of Congress Cataloging-in-Publication Data

Names: Alexander, Gale, 1944- author.
Title: 30 days of hope for joy through a child's severe illness / Gale Alexander.
Other titles: Thirty days of hope for joy through a child's incurable disease
Description: Birmingham : New Hope Publishers, 2016.
Identifiers: LCCN 2016002458 | ISBN 9781596694750 (sc)
Subjects: LCSH: Consolation. | Sick children. | Epidermolysis bullosa--Religious aspects-
-Christianity.
Classification: LCC BV4910.5 .A44 2016 | DDC 242/.4--dc23
LC record available at http://lccn.loc.gov/2016002458

ISBN-10: 1-59669-475-0
ISBN-13: 978-1-59669-475-0

N164115 • 0716 • 2.2M1

TABLE OF CONTENTS

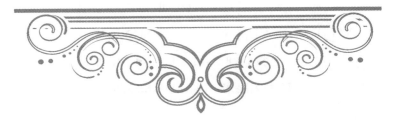

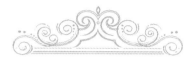

POWERFUL PEOPLE

Foreword
by Becky Rieksts

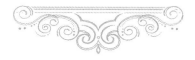

ASHINGTON, DC, is a place where who you know can be one of the most important ingredients for success. Knowing impressive people can supposedly help you get ahead. Over the course of my career, I've had the privilege to be a witness to many important world events and been in the presence of kings, prime ministers, and presidents of the United States. But none of those "important" people of the world have profoundly impacted me in ways that a little girl and her family have over the last seven-plus years.

I will never forget where I was when Joella Gale Murray was born. On June 21, 2007, I was a White House producer for CNN and I was going to spend the day traveling with President George W. Bush to Athens, Alabama, to tour the Browns Ferry Nuclear Plant where he would give a speech on his energy policies. On my way to Andrews Air Force Base, I called her very-soon-to-be-parents, Joe and Katie, to tell them I was praying for them as they headed to the hospital for their scheduled C-section. I boarded Air Force One and went on with my work. In the middle of President Bush's speech, I saw that Joe was calling me so I took the call. I could tell from his voice that things were very serious. Ella's birth had been much more dramatic than anyone could have ever predicted. Ella had an almost immediate diagnosis of epidermolysis bullosa (EB). She is missing a key protein that causes her skin to blister easily. But on that day, I was introduced to one of the strongest people I have ever known. We quickly got to see what a fighter she was.

It's not lost on me that I was following around the most powerful man in the world, and we were at one of the most powerful places on earth on the day of her birth. Brown's Ferry was the first nuclear plant that the United States government opened, and at its opening, it was the largest nuclear facility in the world. But sometimes God chooses to show His power and strength through much smaller people in normal life events. In this case, it was a 7 pound, 4 ounce baby whom God used to show that He answers prayers. All of the Murrays' friends and families were praying hard for Ella during those first few hours when things seemed to be the most critical. She made it through the night with what I truly believe was God's strength and power filling her lungs with each breath. Immediately, the body of Christ came together to minister to the Murrays in every way possible. The Lord really showed Himself to numerous people in those days, and I believe that He received the glory in that situation.

As a friend of Joe and Katie, I have the honor and privilege to see how God works in the life of this precious little girl. Ella continues to be a strong fighter and has blossomed into a smart, creative, curious child. I know she must have her rough moments, but I have always admired her for the way she handles her condition. This awful disease hasn't stopped Ella from doing the things she wants to do. Some activities are modified, but she has always found a way to shine with her interests. She is truly an inspiration to everyone who meets her.

When she was born, Joe and Katie selected John 10:10 as Ella's life verse where Jesus says, "I have come that they may have life, and have it to the full." And Ella is in the process of living life abundantly, despite her skin condition.

A couple of years ago Ella dressed up as a superhero: "Superhero Ella" to be exact. And I can think of no better description for her. She has been used by God since the day she was born to tell of His power and strength working in our lives. She will always be a superhero in my eyes.

BECKY BRITTAN RIEKSTS
Former CNN White House Producer
First Baptist Church, Alexandria, Virginia, Deacon
Ella's Aunt Beck

ACKNOWLEDGEMENTS

F IRST, thank you to Papo Peck and Papo Wance, my grandfathers who held me captive with their stories that taught me to appreciate my heritage and look for adventure in ordinary places. And to my grandmothers, who told and lived the stories of Jesus, making me want to know Him personally.

My Magnolia Sisters, Vickie Cawthra, Linda Stoval, Gretchen Wheeler, and Ebba Stedillie who know that "Telling stories brings people close to us, allowing us to share what it is to be truly human."

Aumi Kauffman Perry who tells stories with oil on canvas, Don Lanum whose unselfishness tells a powerful story, and Sabrina who tells them with a wagging tail.

Thank you to Becky Reiksts, Tori Lane Kovarik, Pastor Don Davidson, and the family of First Baptist Church, Alexandria, Virginia, whose interactions with Ella first inspired this book.

To Curby and Gina Alexander, Val Kulhavy, Pam Creason, Dr. Grant Wilson, Cindy Rogers, and Andrea Mullins who shared encouragement for me to write, and offered constructive help along the way. Thank you to the Rodolph, O'Connell, Peterson, Garbutt, and Hampton families who allowed me to introduce their amazing children.

Thank you to my husband Ron for patiently listening to my stories for 45 years, and to my family who have never discouraged me from following my whims.

Finally, to my muse, Ella, and her parents, Katie and Joe Murray, thank you for your stories of faith, hope, courage, and joy; and for giving us young A. J. whose very existence is a living testimony to those things.

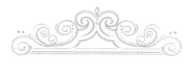

INTRODUCTION

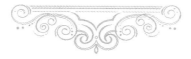

Whereby are given unto us exceeding great and precious promises;
that by these ye might be partakers of the divine nature.

—2 Peter 1:4

It was a hot August afternoon in Casper, Wyoming, and a rare opportunity for Ron and me to take our three, four-year-old grandchildren, Ella, Sam, and Nate, for ice cream. It was "2-for-1 Tuesday" at Johnny J's Diner. If you bought one milkshake, you got the second free. So, we generously invited the parents and great-grandmother Mary to join us.

Seated around the big corner booth, the nine of us studied the flavor options. Each of us ordered something different and delectable. When the milkshakes arrived, complete with a glob of whipped cream and a cherry on top, we each took our first tastes and made comments on the deliciousness of the sweet concoctions. Ella asked me how my chocolate-marshmallow-peanut butter shake tasted. "Simply divine!" was my dramatic answer. The three grandchildren looked at each other then burst into giggles. (I thought it was the sugar.)

"GiGi, what does that word mean? What is divine?" To which I grasped a teachable moment and explained that divine was what you called something when it was the very best you had ever seen or tasted; it was heavenly . . . too good for ordinary words to describe.

For the rest of the visit, all three children liberally practiced their use of the word . . . the scrambled eggs were divine; the cartoon show was double divine; throwing rocks into the river was triple divine. They added a new word to their vocabularies and I added a memory. Because my use of the word divine never failed to bring a smile to the face of a little girl who had lived her entire life grimacing with pain, I used the word often, and I began to call Ella, "Little Miss Divine."

Ella Murray, my daughter's first child, was born with a rare, debilitating genetic disease called epidermolysis bullosa. EB. Only one of every 20,000 babies is born with the disease, and most do not survive to adulthood. EB has been called "the worst disease you've never heard of." Certainly, our family knew nothing of it until Ella was born. We became fast learners and continue to learn about this very rare disease.

Early on, Katie, Joe, and Ella were given immediate support and hope through an organization that helps provide for the practical and emotional needs of EB families. The Dystrophic Epidermolysis Bullosa Research Association, referred to as debra, provides a lifeline by raising money to provide services and promote research for a cure. In a debra newsletter, EB is described like this:

> Epidermolysis Bullosa (EB) is a rare genetic connective tissue disorder. There are many genetic variations, but all share the prominent symptom of extremely fragile skin that blisters and tears from minor friction or trauma. Internal organs and bodily systems can also be seriously

affected by the disease. EB is always painful, often pervasive and debilitating, and is in some cases lethal before the age of 30. EB affects 1 out of 20,000 live births and those born with it are often called "Butterfly Children." There is no treatment or cure.

There is currently no cure for EB. Antiseptic baths, salves, and ointments serve to protect the open sores from infection, and bandages, which can cover 70% of the body, protect the fragile skin from traumatic tearing or blistering.

Fingers and toes often fuse in a way that makes mobility increasingly difficult, holding a pencil impossible, and walking an arduous task. Even eating can cause friction that leads to blistering of the esophagus and strictures in the throat, eventually leading to reliance on a feeding tube for most nutrition.

The Murray family was quickly flooded with gestures of goodwill to help them through this unexpected difficulty. But, as a grandmother, I stood to the side, feeling I must be strong for my daughter and stalwart before the many friends who were watching. I felt alone, helpless, and afraid. My husband suffered in his own way, but the two of us didn't really know how to comfort each other, so we maintained solitary prayer vigils.

Eventually, each of us found our new normal, and were thankful for every sign of hope that sweet Ella would be with us one day more. Katie became a competent and tender caregiver for her daughter, and amazed everyone with her buoyant spirit and nursing skill. Joe stayed the course and completed his law degree, determined to meet his goal to provide well for his family over the long haul. There were daily signs of God's love, mercy, and provision. Our daughter reported on the miraculous progress Ella made, and of the inexplicable goodness being showered on the family of three. They smiled more and cried less as hope booted despair aside. Ron proclaimed confidently to all who asked that a cure for EB would soon be found, and I began to write stories about Little Miss Divine.

My friend Ebba Stedillie helped me to understand why it was important to tell stories when she wrote, "Whether we're struggling with the boulders and ravines of our life's path, whether we're searching for just the right language of comfort or celebrating life's victories, our stories help to give direction, solace, and insight." Jesus used stories and parables to teach life lessons, reveal Himself, and make a personal connection with His followers. Stories continue to allow us, as Ebba says, "to meet on our unique journeys, however briefly, and experience the contented sense of connection, of belonging, or adding our own stories to the single atlas of human experience."

The raw details of childhood afflictions are often difficult to share and even more difficult to hear, but few will turn away from hearing a real life story about a child's triumph over adversity. The stories in this book pay homage to the lives of six children who have incurable diseases, or conditions that make their daily walk challenging for them and their caregivers. Each story is a gift of hope and encouragement for those who love a child who is sick. They tell of how these children, despite a physical, emotional, or cognitive disadvantage, are living life to the full, inspiring the divine goodness in others, and spurring them to acts of uncommon generosity and kindness.

For we are God's masterpiece. He has created us anew in Christ Jesus, so we can do the good things he planned for us long ago.

—Ephesians 2:10

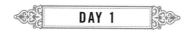

DAY 1

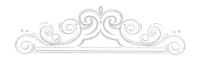

TEAM JOELLA

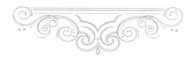

Consider it pure joy, my brothers and sisters, whenever you face trials of many kinds, because you know that the testing of your faith produces perseverance. Let perseverance finish its work so that you may be mature and complete, not lacking anything . . . Blessed is the one who perseveres under trial because, having stood the test, that person will receive the crown of life that the Lord has promised to those who love him.

—JAMES 1:2–4, 12 NIV

WITHIN days after her birth, prayer partners joined hearts around the world. Katie and Joe began a blog to keep thousands of friends, family, and total strangers informed of their baby's condition. Team Joella became the strong right arm of the Murray family. This is the first post on teamjoella.blogspot.com, written by her dad, Joe Murray:

Thank you for visiting Joella Gale Murray's blog site. Katie and I are so blessed to have this little princess in our life despite the tough news that she has a very rare skin disease, epidermolysis bullosa, which only affects 50 out of 1 million births in the United States. We certainly did not expect nor plan for Joella's condition, given that Katie's pregnancy was a textbook one with excellent check-ups and doctor's visits. We believe the amniotic fluid in Katie's uterus protected little Joella all throughout the pregnancy, and it is a miracle she survived being born. We have accepted the fact that God has chosen us to be her parents and will do so to the best of our ability.

Currently, Ella is being cared for at the Children's National Hospital in Washington, DC, by some of the best doctors in the world. The main form of treatment is to keep her skin hydrated and to keep her blisters on her extremities from contracting any infections. At this point, her vital signs are terrific. Her little heart and lungs are working beautifully; it's just her skin, the largest organ, which is impacted by the disease.

Katie and I visit her daily and watch her move, open her eyes periodically, and pray for God's healing and comfort. She is in a general state of pain all over her little body. The pain is being managed by morphine and other pain medications. She recognizes her mommy and daddy's voices and moves to show us she knows we are there.

At this time, Katie and I understand that each day we have with her is a gift from above. The good Lord could take her home at any time, but also could allow her to have a full life with treatment. We just don't know. There is no cure for the disease at this time, yet research for a cure is encouraging.

What we do know is that we have grown tremendously in the knowledge that God is in complete control of Joella's, Katie's, and my life. The Holy Spirit is sustaining us with the comfort of hundreds, if not thousands, of praying folks all over the world showering kind words and encouragement. We understand this news is very hard to digest and that folks want to help us in any tangible way they can. All we need and ask for at this time is prayer for Joella's condition to improve and that she would be able to have a productive life free from pain.

I close this post with a few Bible Scripture verses that have been impactful to Katie and me since Joella's birth. Thank you for all your love.

And we know that in all things God works for the good of those who love him, who have been called according to his purpose.

—Romans 8:28 NIV

Many are the plans in a person's heart, but it is the Lord's purpose that prevails.

—Proverbs 19:21 NIV

The prayer of a righteous person is powerful and effective.

—James 5:16 NIV

You will keep in perfect peace those whose minds are steadfast, because they trust in you.

—Isaiah 26:3 NIV

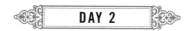

DAY 2

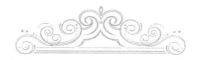

CELEBRATION

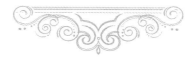

When you see these things, your heart will rejoice.
You will flourish like the grass! Everyone will see the LORD's hand
of blessing on his servants.

—ISAIAH 66:14

T<small>HESE</small> are the words of Congressman Joe Wilson (SC-02) on the floor of the United States House of Representatives on Monday, July 23, 2007:

> Madam Speaker, today, I am happy to congratulate Joseph and Kathryn Murray of Alexandria, Virginia, on the birth of their beautiful baby girl. Joella "Ella" Gale Murray was born on Thursday, June 21, 2007, at 1:03 pm weighing 7 pounds, 4 ounces and measuring 19 inches long. Ella has been born into a loving home, where she will be raised by parents who are devoted to her well-being and bright future. Her birth is a blessing.

Ella's birth was celebrated by this announcement placed into the Congressional Record of the United States House of Representatives. (Joe worked for Congressman Wilson when Ella was born.) As I read it, I thought of how the birth of Jesus Christ was celebrated by those of both high and lowly station: kings, angels, and shepherds. Ella's birth was acknowledged by Congressmen, family, friends, and total strangers all around the world. Just as Mary was not exactly sure what lay ahead for her infant son, none of us were certain of Ella's future. Nevertheless, we celebrated.

When discussing baby names, Joe and Katie decided to name a boy Alexander . . . Katie's maiden name. Because the name means "defender of men," it was appropriate for the son of a lawyer/politician. A girl would be named Joella Gale for her great-grandmother with Jo added to honor her dad and Gale to identify with her mother and me. The name Joella was new to us, but research shows it to be the female derivative of

Joel, which means, "Jehovah is God." Our granddaughter had a strong name, but we had no way of understanding just how strong she would prove herself to be.

Early each morning in the weeks following Ella's birth, her daddy grabbed his Bible, doffed a red baseball cap that read "Rookie Dad" and left for the Children's National Hospital in Washington, DC, to check on his daughter and to participate in her bandage change. Every person dealing with this baby was a "Rookie" because no one, not even the professionals in the NICU, had ever before dealt directly with this disease.

There was a lot of experimenting with her care. Each time a new technique with feeding or bandages worked, there was celebration. When she opened her eyes and looked steadily into the eyes of her mother, there was celebration. When she pulled the feeding tube out of her nose all by herself, and nursed from a bottle, there was celebration. When she responded to an image in the mirror and a music maker placed inside her incubator, there was celebration. When her parents could hold and rock her, in spite of tubes and a bulky sheepskin mat, there was celebration. And when, 33 days after her birth, she went home with her parents, there was celebration.

From the very beginning, Ella seemed to draw strength from her name. Even though she never got to know her great-grandmother, she models Big Mama's resolute courage and has demonstrated in countless ways that Jehovah is God. She understands that her Heavenly Father celebrates her life and knows who she is just as, "He counts the stars and calls them all by name" (Psalm 147:4).

I like to think that the members gathered in the chambers of the House of Representatives the day Ella's birth announced took a breath, and a moment to glance away from the business of government to celebrate the miracle of birth and new beginnings. God, the author of life, celebrates when we acknowledge these miracles of His making. By celebrating moments of grace in the midst of turmoil and stress, we applaud His gifts of life, love, and hope.

Pageant, praise, parade
Accolades, applause, awards
Give gladness to good

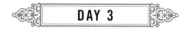

DAY 3

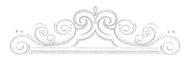

YOU MUST HAVE BEEN
A BEAUTIFUL BABY

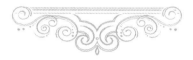

Children are a gift from the LORD; they are a reward from him.

—PSALM 127:3

On September 19, 2007, at First Baptist Church, Alexandria, Virginia, Ella's parents took their three-month-old daughter forward during the morning worship service and dedicated her to the Lord. In his weekly online journal, Pastor Don Davidson reflected on the event:

> Not to be confused with infant baptism, or 'Christening,' [dedication] is a meaningful few moments at the altar where parents commit themselves to raising their child in a Christian home, teaching Jesus' ways, and modeling before that little one the ways to follow Him. The baby won't remember any of it, and will one day, when older, have to make her own commitment to the Lord. It doesn't happen automatically, because God honors the free will that He gave us, but it is almost inevitable when those parents honor the vows made in that service. Just a few years later, down the aisle the child comes and into the baptistery . . . and I get to hold him again.
>
> [During the dedication] I get to hold the baby, speak Scripture into little ears, and present him to his new family of faith at First Baptist Church. These children are animated, usually bright-eyed, and they almost never cry while I'm holding them. I think each baby is the most beautiful baby I have ever seen.
>
> Yesterday was no exception—but what an exceptional moment it was! Joe and Katie Murray brought forward their little girl, Joella, to be presented to God. She's the baby born this summer with a very rare skin disorder

that made us fear we'd not get to keep her very long. And so we all prayed, deacons ministered in every way imaginable, and Bible Fellowship friends brought meals every night to the weary parents and sets of grandparents.

[Joe and Katie] see her as a special gift from God (as we all do now) and on Sunday they were powerfully and publicly giving her back to Him, for whatever His will might be in the future. It is possible to trust our good and loving heavenly Father—even with that which is most precious to us. You learn that, over time and through dark valleys.

Baby Joella and I were at a cookout together on Saturday night, so we did a little "bonding" and practicing for the big event. We were both pretty confident on Sunday morning. And the service went off beautifully.

Later, during the choir music . . . Joella did break down and let out a wail or two. There are times when that is rather distracting to me and takes away from my worship experience—but not yesterday. A big smile came across my face as I realized how wonderful babies and life really are. Their arrival on the scene means that God has not yet given up on His world. That there is still some great thing to be done, and maybe this one will do it.

Ours for just a while
To raise and love and cherish
God's now and forever

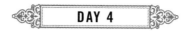

DAY 4

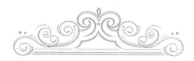

CALEB'S REACH

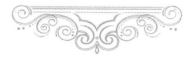

I will refine them like silver and purify them like gold.

—ZECHARIAH 13:9

WITH outstretched arms and a wide grin, he toddled toward the enticement of a shiny silver dollar that I held in my hand. It was right before his first birthday, and Caleb took his first steps in my kitchen. After all, I introduced his parents to each other and arranged their first date. In my memory of Caleb as a baby, he was always smiling and always eagerly reaching out for something. His first spoken word was "ball," and he reached for any he saw. He was a golden boy, loved and adored by all who knew him.

Just two months after that first step, Caleb was taken to Denver Children's Hospital where cancer was removed from his spine, and it was a very long time before he walked again. The diagnosis was neuroblastoma and malignant neoplasm of other sites. Later, as a direct result of treatment for this rare cancer, Caleb was forced to reach even farther when he was diagnosed with opsoclonus-myoclonus syndrome with specific and unspecified mental disorders. For most of his life, Caleb has had to stretch and reach for things many thought would be forever beyond his grasp.

Now a young adult with an IQ in the borderline range, verbal abilities below average, and impaired perceptual reasoning, Caleb continues to struggle. Nevertheless, he has that same radiant smile, and the quality of this young man's life is not found in his limitations, but in the magnitude of his reach. Determination, hard work, courage, bravery, and perseverance have made him his mom's hero. He is his dad's valued, irreplaceable partner in several business and hunting ventures. His three siblings say he is the best big brother in the world. And when, as a teenager, he prayed to ask Jesus to be the Lord and Savior of the life he had been given to live, Caleb reached for and claimed the greatest gift of all.

Reaching through and beyond trials is part of the refining process that purifies our faith. Writing to struggling Christians in the northern Roman provinces that are now known as Turkey, Peter urged his readers to endure their suffering as refinement of their faith. "It is being tested as fire tests and purifies gold—though your faith is far more precious than mere gold" (1 Peter 1:7).

Reaching beyond his expected capabilities is what Caleb does. It's what those who care for a sick child do. It's what we all do when we strive for the calling God puts on our lives. We reach beyond our capabilities, proving that we trust Him.

A bad ice and wind storm ravaged the trees in our town one spring. The large cottonwood in our yard was torn asunder, so an arborist was called to trim and save the grand tree. I stood at the door nervously watching a young man climb precariously to the top of the swaying limbs, pruning tools in hand and safety rope around his waist. On the ground below was his spotter—a strong, confident guy who intently held the safety ropes taunt in upstretched fists. It was Caleb. No longer a baby reaching for a silver dollar, or a teenager reaching to comprehend mathematic equations, but a man reaching out to protect and help another. That prize is more than silver. It's pure gold.

Hands and heart outstretched
Treasure beyond common grasp
Reach far; joy ahead!

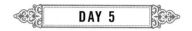

DAY 5

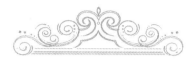

FREE FALLING

He does great things too marvelous to understand.
He performs countless miracles.

—JOB 9:10

Now, jump!" My young feet were planted on the edge of the hayloft in my grandfather's barn. He stood below with outstretched arms. It was a long way down but my Papo Peck was big and strong. With absolute confidence that he would catch me, I jumped. For a split second I experienced the miracle of free falling . . . I flew knowing I would land safely in the strong arms of my Papo . . . and I did.

Skydiving has never been on my bucket list. You couldn't pay me to jump out of an airplane and freefall into thin air. No way! But free falling into life, knowing that my Heavenly Father stands with outstretched arms to catch me, has been my way of living ever since I asked Jesus to be the Lord of my life. Just as a skydiver bounces among the clouds during a free fall, a child of God bounces with faith-filled confidence from one miracle to another. Paul says in Galatians 3:5, "Does God give you the Holy Spirit and work miracles among you because you obey the law? Of course not! It is because you believe the message you heard about Christ." We free fall because we trust.

A happening that can only be attributed to divine intervention is called miraculous. With a desperately sick child, miracles are often all that get a family from one day to the next. In our case, the first miracle came when a late-term ultrasound showed that the baby Katie had carried so effortlessly was in breech position with one foot firmly lodged in the birth canal. A C-section was scheduled. Three grandparents from out of state were present for the birth. The breech position and C-section most likely saved Ella's life, and three grandparents were near to give the emotional and physical support that was needed. Some would say "lucky coincidences," but we said "miracles."

In the days immediately after her birth, many people prayed for Ella's complete miraculous healing. Katie and Joe's church even held a special prayer meeting where 200 people knelt together to intervene on her behalf and to lift our family in petitions for grace and mercy. Complete healing has been granted to others in dire circumstances, but Ella wasn't instantaneously healed and sent home as a healthy baby with perfect, flawless skin. Her miracles came in the form of events that could only be explained as divine intervention.

We slept well at night. Nourishing, home cooked meals were delivered to the house each afternoon for over a month. Money to pay for gasoline and parking for the daily trips to the hospital was given. Joe became knowledgeable in assisting the nurses with the daily bandage change. Katie became more confident and hopeful as she spent time researching the disease on the Internet and learning from other EB moms. (Such technology is a special brand of miracle!) Ella's own tiny hand pulled the feeding tube out of her nose and she began to nurse from a bottle and gain weight.

A work friend of Joe's vaguely remembered hearing that a friend of a friend who lived in Atlanta, Georgia, had a child with EB. He contacted Andrew Tavani who immediately called Joe and came to Alexandria to offer Joe and Katie encouragement and hope for Ella's future. This visit was a turning point . . . a miracle . . . in their attitude about their daughter's prospects.

debra of America (Dystrophic Epidermolysis Bullosa Research Association) is a nonprofit organization whose mission is to support families with EB and provide funds for research for a cure for this, "Worst disease you've never heard of." Within hours of Ella's birth, Katie and Joe were contacted by this organization that sped to provide every level of support. The mother of a baby who did not survive EB came to Alexandria from Kentucky and spent a weekend helping the Murrays prepare their small apartment and readjust their lives to care for their baby. Good things continue to flow through debra to this day.

Miracles come both from God's own hand, and from His hand on the hearts and hands of others. Ella's life is a testimony to both varieties. Her parents don't discount any intervention that can only be explained as His divine love for our girl and the plan He has for her life. At times they are stunned at the wonder of it all and ask, like David, "Who can list the glorious miracles of the LORD? Who can ever praise him enough?" (Psalm 106:2). This family free falls from miracle to miracle. Often the fall takes their breath away. They always know there are strong arms outstretched, ready to catch them, so they jump.

Fearing the unknown
Frozen on the precipice
Freedom's in the fall

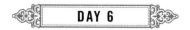

DAY 6

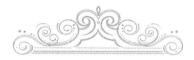

WEE WARRIORS

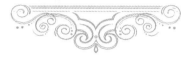

Then he took the children in his arms and placed his hands on their heads and blessed them.

—MARK 10:16

Ask your children and grandchildren to pray. Tell them about Ella and how God is listening to their prayers." So many people prayed for Ella soon after her birth and beyond. Anytime someone would say, "we are praying for Ella," I always requested them to ask their children to pray, and tell them that their prayers are heard.

I believe there is something about the simple, sincere prayers of a child that cuts through the drone of ordinary prayer, going to the head of the line and straight to God's ear. Because of this, I want children to pray very specifically for Ella's needs. By so praying, their little hearts will be made more sensitive to the needs of people around them.

- Callie prays that Ella would not have so many boo-boos.
- Estelle prays she will get a lot of money so she can pay doctors to find a cure for EB.
- Ethan prays to be the doctor who will find that cure.
- Sam prays that one day his cousin will be able to run and play with him.
- Nate prays that Ella will have "good joy."
- Elsa, Anya, and Hans pray that she will be healthy.

Part of our responsibility as parents and grandparents is to teach our little ones of both the love of God and the power of prayer. The psalmist admonished us, "Tell the next generation about the glorious deeds of the Lord, about his power and his mighty wonders" (Psalm 78:4). Wee Prayer Warriors grow in faith and trust as they experience answered prayer.

Beyond this, a praying child learns to show empathy and be less self-centered. As Paul urged, they, "rejoice with those who rejoice, weep with those who weep" (Romans 12:15 ESV). Praying for the troubles of another makes it more likely that the child will transfer caring into real life acts of kindness. In Ella's case, some children she plays with slow their pace so she can keep up, help her to carry her books, are very protective of her, and are just a little more mindful of being gentle than with their other playmates. I've seen them at her side at school and church and these Wee Warriors make me proud.

We seem to want to shield our children from the raw reality of disease, poverty, abuse, crime, and neglect. Maybe we think they can't handle the truth of life. Maybe we adults can't handle not having the answers to their questions about such injustice. Guiding our children and grandchildren to pray very specifically for a hurting child will position them to love unconditionally and without judgment.

Tiny little prayers
Float above the heavy din
Finding God's own ear

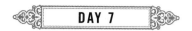

DAY 7

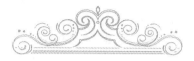

LEGACY OF SERVICE

*For we are God's masterpiece. He has created us anew in Christ
Jesus, so we can do the good things he planned for us long ago.*

—EPHESIANS 2:10

A BEDRAGGLED, homeless man made his way across the parking lot of the grocery store where Katie was loading bags of groceries into their minivan. Ella was seated inside and watched with attentive curiosity as the raggedly dressed man asked her mom for money.

"I can't give you money," Katie said "but I'll share my food with you." The man said he needed money, not food, and walked away.

Back in the car, Ella told her mom they should give the man the Manna Bag she had prepared at her girls' missions group a few weeks earlier. The bag was a gallon size ziplock bag containing a toothbrush and toothpaste, a pair of new white socks, a comb, a bag of peanuts, small cups of applesauce and pudding, plastic spoon, beef jerky, crackers and peanut butter, and of course, a Bible tract. Driving toward the man who was walking across the parking lot, Katie slowed the car, lowered the window just enough to hand the bag to the man and said, "My daughter wants you to have this." The stranger took the bag, and as he examined the contents, his face softened. "Thank you, little girl, and God bless."

When Ella told me the story, I quoted, *"When you do it to the least, you've done it to me.* Do you know what that means, Ella?" She answered, "Giving food to a hungry man makes Jesus happy, but it makes me happy, too."

When you help others, you help yourself. I first learned this important truth from my two grandmothers when I accompanied them to weekly meetings of the Woman's Missionary Circle in their small country churches. I saw the fervor, pride, and joy with which they planned ways to minister to the less fortunate.

When I was a young preteen girl, my parents volunteered to help start a church in a rapidly growing new section of my hometown. A lovely lady, Miss Charlene, joined the small congregation and announced that she wanted to begin a group called GAs . . . Girl's Auxiliary. I was in! We met every Wednesday night in a tiny nook at the back of the storefront building, which was our church. My eyes and heart were opened to the world beyond my small hometown. Learning to care about the needs of others motivated me to become a stronger young Christian.

Years later, I had a daughter of my own, but a church that did not provide missions education for children. So, I started a group of GAs . . . Girls in Action (times had changed, and so had the name). My daughter Katie was born to be a GA. Everything about the organization took root in her soul. Each Wednesday she brought three or four girls home from school for a snack, then on to church for GAs. What fun it was to be a GA leader and watch my daughter's heart grow eager to share the love of Christ with her friends.

Next came Ella. Because of her physical limitations, it was difficult for her to be involved in the typical childhood activities such as dancing, soccer, or piano lessons. But the minute she was of the right age, Katie enrolled her in GAs at their church. From the first meeting, Ella was taken by the challenge of missions. She came out of each meeting talking about what she learned of the needs of people in her community and around the world. In GAs she learned that other children in the world had needs that made her disease seem less isolating. GAs helped her to know that she is not alone in her need.

By giving a Manna Bag to a poor stranger, Ella learned that she can be a missionary from her seat in the family van. This small gesture was as important to the kingdom of God as traveling across the ocean to minister in faraway lands.

God doesn't measure the miles traveled or the magnitude of a ministry. He measures the magnitude of a heart.

Ella comes from a line of strong, confident women who knew that self-esteem grows through giving a little more of ourselves, being a little less self-centered, and trying a little more each day to help others. She's doing a good job with the legacy of service that has been passed down to her. Individually and collectively, we would all benefit from such a legacy.

> *Stoop down and grow tall*
> *Sharing makes a larger self*
> *Giving grows giver*

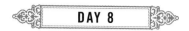

DAY 8

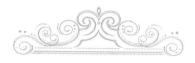

WALKING WITH SCHUYLER

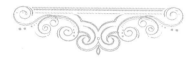

As iron sharpens iron, so a friend sharpens a friend.

—Proverbs 27:17

FIVE young mothers meet at the local coffee shop. The hour spent together twice a month is for respite, encouragement, prayer, praise, and to sharpen one another's faith and resilience to be the mom God expects her to be. Each woman has a child with a physical or cognitive exception to the norm.

On one particular Monday, praise and thanksgiving displaced weariness and discouragement. Schuyler had taken her first steps alone. Defying medical prediction, she stood alone, on her own two feet, and took a couple of unassisted steps toward her father's outstretched arms. Then was prompted to take more steps to her mother. Schuyler, with squeals of excitement, continued to walk back and forth to her parents. This was truly a special blessing to her family, including her grandparents who were in town visiting. She was almost five and a half years old and on her way toward disclaiming the naysaying that surrounded her birth.

As they awaited the arrival of their second daughter, Cecie and Blake outfitted the nursery, prepared a two and a half year old for the intrusion of a sibling, and braced themselves to receive a baby with an undiagnosed genetic anomaly. Prenatal tests indicated an irregularity but no clear expectations of the outcome. Schuyler was born with a rare chromosome disorder, so rare that her parents call it "Schuyler Syndrome."

No one knew just how this unknown condition would manifest. Would she walk? Talk? Feed and dress herself? Read? Function independently? Have reasonable cognitive capabilities? Her parents didn't know what to expect, but they knew one thing—God gave them this daughter to love, care for, and guide toward her full potential.

Hope for the walk they faced came in Isaiah 40:31, "But they that wait upon the LORD shall renew their strength; they shall mount up with wings as eagles; they shall run, and not be weary; and they shall walk, and not faint" (KJV). This family did a lot of waiting for Schuyler's first solo steps, and their faith needed a lot of renewing.

Now Schuyler, with the aid of ankle orthotics, walks and even runs. She rides the bus to school, has a nonverbal vocabulary, and one step at a time, the other things doctors said not to expect of her are loosening their grip on her quality of life. Her family is realistically optimistic about her future. When I visit my daughter's family, I always look forward to Wednesday night fellowship dinner at First Baptist, Alexandria, Virginia. Schuyler, sporting a large, colorful bow in her hair, walks to the table her family shares with the Murrays. She enjoys her food and listens to the chatter of others at the table. When the meal is over, she walks to children's choir where she participates as an appreciative listener, and when it's over, she walks, smiling, into her mother's waiting arms. Schuyler's heart can sing, "You have kept my feet from slipping. So now I can walk in your presence, O God, in your life-giving light" (Psalm 56:13).

For Cecie, the group of moms who meet bimonthly are iron sharpening iron. These women understand the importance of renewed strength and how significant one tiny step can be. Even a sword of the finest steel needs honing. Slaying our personal dragons demands a sharp sword. The iron of faith, family, and friends fortify us to do battle!

Climbing a mountain
Each step a triumph of faith
Summit view is sharp

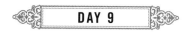

DAY 9

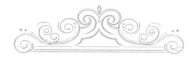

LETTER OF HOPE

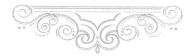

*You yourselves are our letter, written on our hearts,
known and read by everyone.*

—2 Corinthians 3:2 NIV

T HREE-YEAR-OLD Ella was ready for preschool, but it was evident that she would need a personal assistant to help her navigate outside the safe haven of her home. Deciding whether or not to make this big step was very difficult for the Murray family. They wanted their daughter to experience more of her world and make friends her own age, but they were concerned about how she would manage in an active school environment. They didn't imagine that Ella would become the teacher in her school.

Miss Tori is a beautiful young artist who worked as assistant teacher in Ella's preschool class. For one year she patiently guided the shy little girl to and from the playground, helped her to manage her backpack, and led her through the halls of the huge First Baptist Church of Alexandria, Virginia, where the preschool was housed. Her mission was to be sure Ella was included in every activity, and that she never sat in the shadows simply watching the other children.

Tori helped to make preschool a resounding success and Ella blossomed. When summer came, this sensitive artist organized an Art Camp for children, and Ella was the first child she invited to participate. It was Ella's first day camp. What fun they all had with paper, paint, and brushes!

At the end of pre-K, Ella was ready for public school kindergarten. Ron and I attended her preschool graduation ceremony, where the only person more proud than the parents and grandparents was Miss Tori. She beamed as Ella walked, with very little assistance, across the stage to receive her diploma, and she was the first to claim a hug from the new graduate.

With preschool successfully completed, Tori's services as an aide were no longer needed. She sent a letter of thanks to Katie and Joe for allowing her to be part of Ella's life and to share her personal story of what Ella had taught her. She revealed that depression, addiction, and shame resulting from sexual trauma had taken hold of her life. Many days the sadness could only be born through the emotional outlet of painting, writing, and immersing herself in the happy play of children at the preschool.

Realizing she needed help, Tori went to a women's retreat designed for victims of sexual trauma. She connected with a wise mentor who suggested that whenever the despair was more than she thought she could bear, she should focus on a mental image of someone who exemplified courage and peace in the face of pain and hopelessness. Tori told her mentor about a little girl named Ella.

She wrote, "Ella loved me as a teacher and as a person. She saw something in me that was worth loving and trusting, and I wasn't going to call Ella a liar. I had no reason to mistrust her and would never want to hurt her. So, I had to fight for myself, for my own healing, if not for my own sake, for Ella's because I trusted and loved her."

The letter of hope that this young woman needed was written on a small face. Ella's patience and resolve through difficulty increased Tori's faith that hope was also there for her. Our lives are letters for those in our circle of influence to read. A desperate soul who is losing ground should be able to read our letter and see hope written there.

Ella and Tori remain fast friends . . . texting and enjoying each other's company whenever possible. However, Tori's life is much different from when they met on that first day of preschool. No longer chained to her past, Tori works with victims of sexual trauma, connecting them to resources and support systems, shedding light on issues often clothed in silence. She has become a recognized artist in Northern Virginia, published several books of poetry, and was designated Poet Laureate of Alexandria City in 2013. One of her best poems is about a little girl who helped her to find a path out of her dark place. As a speaker and educator she helps churches and organizations to design programs for helping those who come through their doors with needs for healing. Now a new bride with a promising future, her life is a letter of hope.

Spoken with silence
Words of hope need not be loud
Message sent by being

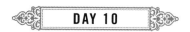

DAY 10

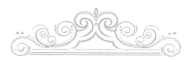

PURSUED BY A PUP

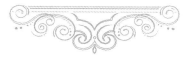

For the Son of Man came to seek and save those who are lost.

—Luke 19:10

MY GRANDDAUGHTER is not demanding. She never asks for much. Even at Christmas, her wish list is short and simple. One of the few things Ella ever asked for was a puppy. When she was a toddler, her favorite place to go was the pet store at the mall where she would sit in her stroller and gaze longingly at the doggies in the window. Her first spoken word was "dog," and her first request in her nightly prayers was for God to give her one.

For a child with EB, having a pet of any kind can be risky. Small, sharp claws and teeth, not to mention rough play, can be disastrous to fragile skin. We tried to pacify our granddaughter with a lifelike stuffed animal. "Doggie" filled the need for a while, but the request for a real, live puppy never went away. Ella really wanted a dog.

Finally, after three years of prayers by Ella, research by her parents, and conferring with other EB families about the wisdom of having a dog, Katie, Joe, and Ella began the search. Every Saturday morning they visited animal shelters in their area and looked for the dog that met all their criteria: smallish, non-shedding, docile, kid-friendly.

After several disappointing searches, the family decided to be at the nearby animal shelter when the doors opened on one special Saturday morning. They wanted to be the first to look at the adoptable dogs. There in a cage at the back of the room was a litter of four Cockapoo puppies! Joe pointed to the one who made eye contact with him and told the attendant, "We want that one."

"Not so fast," said the attendant. "You might want her, but we have to see if she wants you." The Murrays were instructed to go to a private room and wait to meet this prospective new member of their family. Katie and Joe stood quietly against the back wall. Ella sat expectantly in the middle of the floor. When Sabrina was brought into the room (yes, her name really was, and still is, Sabrina) she did all the normal puppy things. She sniffed feet and the box of toys, looked suspiciously at the new humans, chased her tail a bit, and then she saw Ella sitting in the floor. She stopped, cocked her head once, and ever so slowly and softly padded toward the little girl. She lay down close to Ella's side, put her head in Ella's lap, and lay totally still while Ella stroked her silky ears.

Katie looked at Joe and said, "Well, I guess we found our new family member."

I have heard Jesus Christ referred to as the Hound of Heaven because He so faithfully tracks us down until he gets our attention and makes us His own. One of the most beloved Bible verses is Psalm 23:6 where David avows, "Surely your goodness and unfailing love will pursue me all the days of my life, and I will live in the house of the LORD forever." It's a comfort to know He never gives up the hunt. Knowing how Sabrina chose Ella, and how she has to this very day been at her side as the most gentle, loyal, and protective of companions, I cherish the gift of being pursued by One who loves us and longs to stay by our side through the good and bad of life.

Pursuing answers
I am pursued by His love
Pup chasing its tail?

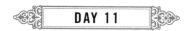

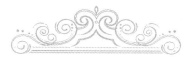

PORTRAIT OF PEACE

For he himself is our peace.

—Ephesians 2:14 NIV

KATIE and Aumi have been friends since their preteen days. The quiet, gentle spirits of Aumi and her sister Osa comforted my daughter through many teenage dramas.

Aumi Kauffman Perry is an artist. Her oil paintings have gained worldwide attention and grace the walls of many homes and art galleries. While still life subjects are her hallmark, I am partial to her portraits. She is able to capture the true spirit of her subjects—their essence—on canvas for all time. To see into the spirit of a subject, no other medium could ever replace the transcendent quality of a really fine oil portrait.

When Ella was four years old and on a visit to our town, Katie and Aumi arranged a play date with her and Aumi's two daughters, Elsa and Anja. The two young moms chatted, sipped tea, and watched the three little girls engage in unusually calm, sweet, peaceful play. Later, Aumi asked if she could paint a portrait of Ella. She saw something in Ella's countenance and demeanor that she wanted to put on canvas.

Only a few weeks later, the painting had been completed with, as the artist put it, "unusual speed and joy." I received the phone call to come to Aumi's studio to see the final product. What I saw on her easel took my breath away. There in delicate pink and white was my precious granddaughter—bandages, scars, and all—holding a butterfly in her disfigured fingers. The picture radiated peace and beauty.

Tormented, restless souls pass close to us as they search for a tranquil spot, a calming touch, a soothing voice, or a moment of repose. Worry and stressful life events can rob our peace. Discontent fuels bitterness and angry intolerance. Even the Children of Israel went through more than a few turbulent periods. Isaiah urged the people of Judah to calm down; "will you be saved. . . in quietness and confidence is your strength" (Isaiah 30:15).

Aumi captured what we have always hoped others would see in Ella: God's calming hand on her life in spite of pain and an uncertain future. Her painting and her life are portraits of God's peace.

Calm and constant gaze
Show the character inside
Artist's brush paints truth

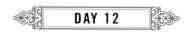

DAY 12

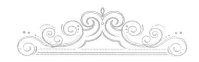

A LITTLE SUGAR

Kind words are like honey—sweet to the soul and healthy for the body.

—Proverbs 16:24

B Y ANY standard, Don is a tough guy. He's tall, tan, toned, and tattooed. He's a body builder, and his muscles are impressive . . . think Rambo meets Mr. Clean! Body building coach/personal fitness trainer by profession, he walks and talks with confidence. He rides a Harley-Davidson. He's a tough guy.

On a Sunday morning as he stood, mug of coffee in hand, gazing out his front window, Don saw his neighbor, Joe, walking hand in hand with his small daughter. She carefully took tiny steps at her daddy's side. The stiff, labored walk was in contrast to the pretty ruffled dress and saucy hair bow she wore. The tough guy softened at the sight. That afternoon he went to the Murray home and offered his help to make that walk a little lighter.

Now each Saturday morning, Joe and Ella walk down the street to the fitness studio where he has customized a workout routine to help Ella build muscle strength, flexibility, and balance. She rings the doorbell, and there he stands with a big smile on his burly face. "There's my girl," he says with arms outstretched. "I need some sugar." Without hesitation, Ella walks into Don's strong arms and places a soft, sweet, innocent kiss on his cheek. Theirs is an unlikely friendship based on shared need and genuine affection. They see each other through unfiltered lenses.

Tough guys are all around us. Some are bullies who use their toughness as a weapon to intimidate and control. For others, a wall of toughness puts space between them and those who would hurt. Toughness can be a façade to hide a vulnerable, seeking soul who yearns for a gentle touch.

In truth, the toughness in each of us occasionally needs a little sugar. A small bit of kindness can make life more palatable, and add renewed energy to our daily walk. A dose of pure, unrefined sweetness could be just the thing to tenderize even the toughest heart.

Frail and fierce define
Keep others at a distance
Sweetness brings them close

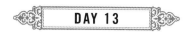
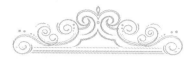

RECIPE FOR BREAD

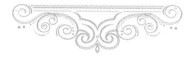

Our Father, which art in heaven, Hallowed be thy name.
Thy kingdom come, Thy will be done in earth as it is in heaven.
Give us this day our daily bread. And forgive us our debts, as we
forgive our debtors. And lead us not into temptation, but deliver
us from evil: For thine is the kingdom, and the power, and
the glory, forever. Amen.

—Matthew 6: 9–13 KJV

P RAYER is part of my spiritual DNA. For as long as I can remember, I have begun each day with "Good morning, LORD," and ended the day with, "Amen." In between has been a steady conversation of adoration, confession, thanks, and supplication. I keep a prayer journal, teach classes on prayer, and identify praying as one of my spiritual gifts.

When Ella was born, I didn't know how to pray.

The supplication part of prayer is awkward for me. I find it difficult to know just what to ask God for. If I pray big, it seems presumptuous to think God would possibly answer such large prayers from such an insignificant person. So, I generally pray small, thinking that if I take the leap and pray grandiose prayers, I have set myself up for disappointment.

As we faced the painful reality of Ella's future, prayers on her behalf were raised by hundreds of voices. For me, it seemed too much to ask for instant, complete healing from EB. After all, if we believe the Bible when it says that God knit us together in our mothers' wombs, and loves us just as we are, then we should accept that God always knew Ella had EB. Even if He didn't intentionally join the two recessive genes that gave her that horrible disease—He knew from conception that she had it. So, if this incurable disease was intended to be her fate, should we contradict and pray for complete healing, or should we pray for other things?

Finally, it dawned on me that the prayer found in Matthew 6:9–13 gave the direction I sought. In this Model Prayer the only supplication is for "our daily bread." The rest of the prayer is about acknowledging God as Lord and trusting Him to lead, guide, direct, and sustain us.

Two directives from the prayer got our family through the early dark days and continue to lead us to find joy in our journey with sweet Ella. We know beyond doubt that God is the Lord of her life and that she is complete and perfect in His eyes, and we know He will provide daily bread for her family.

Even though we never knew the exact content of their prayers, we knew for sure that the Team Joella Prayer Warriors were on the job. Daily bread came when Ella would experience a few hours without pain or there would be a beautiful patch of unmarred skin . . . a feast for the eyes. Or she would enjoy an entire bottle without a new blister forming on her tongue. Someone would suggest a salve that lessened the tormenting itching that plagued her. There were slices of time each day when Joe and Katie were able to simply revel in the joy of their baby girl and completely forgot the EB.

Ron and I would say to each other, "It could be so much worse," and we gave credit to the faithfully uttered supplications that provided daily bread.

As Ella grew stronger and eventually was allowed to go home to be with her parents, we saw loaves of tangible evidence that daily bread was being provided for her and her parents.

A beautiful, kind, competent Ethiopian nurse named Metti was hired to tend to the daily care of Ella so that Katie could have respite from these tasks and continue to be the primary wage earner for the family while Joe completed his law degree. Both Katie and Joe were provided with new and better jobs with flexible work hours and in closer proximity to home. Most importantly, both were inspired with the nursing skills to effectively manage Ella's wound care and bandage changes.

The time came that they knew Katie should quit her job to stay at home full time with Ella. They knew it would be difficult to manage their financial needs on one income, so they designed a "bare bones budget" and prayed simply for their daily bread. From then to now, the Murray breadbasket has been filled.

Life is a complicated journey. If we think too much on the complexity, most of us would throw our hands up in defeat. Sometimes we pray for too much and often for too little. The Lord's Prayer doesn't say, "Give us this day a banquet table filled with everything our hearts desire." Instead, He promises to give us our daily bread . . . just a simple slice of exactly what we need in a specific moment of time.

Hope, faith, love, and prayer
Ingredients for living
Recipe for bread

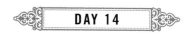

DAY 14

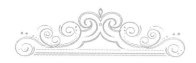

PLANNING FOR
THE PLAN

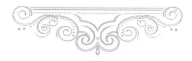

Whether you turn to the right or to the left, your ears will hear a voice behind you, saying, "This is the way; walk in it."

—Isaiah 30:21 NIV

I FIRST heard "God's plan for your life" talked about in GAs . . . Girls Auxiliary, it was called then (now Girls in Action). The realization that my Heavenly Father had a job that could only be done by me was quite a boost to my self-confidence. At age ten, I would lie in bed at night and try to imagine just what that job would be.

Ella raised this question with her daddy when she was six, about the time she began to realize that her disease set her apart from most other children. She asked her parents to explain why she was the only one of her friends who had EB and why God didn't answer her nightly prayer for new skin.

Joe answered something like this: "I think God has a very special plan for your life that requires you to have EB." After that, Ella's questions were not about her disease. They were about that plan! She wanted to know what the plan was, how God was going to tell her what it was, when she should get started on it, and how she should prepare. After several lengthy bedtime discussions on God's plan for Ella, Joe suggested that she begin to pray specifically for God to tell her what the plan was. By deferring responsibility to a higher authority, Joe thought he was off the hook. Not so. This tactic only introduced a whole new set of questions: How will He tell me? Will He whisper in my ear? Will He tell you and then you'll tell me? Will He send me a letter? Will I get a phone call? Ella is a very literal thinker. To tell her there's a job God wants her to do means, "Let's get started!" Thankfully, Joe is a very godly and patient daddy.

Several nights after she was urged to pray for an answer, Ella said, "Daddy, sometimes God gives you a quick answer when you pray, but sometimes He says you have to wait because it isn't the right time. When it's time for me to do my special job, God will let me know."

Job, in his afflictions, was like Ella. He longed to know the divine why and how. It took a long time and multiple losses before he saw that God and His purposes are supreme. Finally he said, "I know that you can do all things; no purpose of yours can be thwarted . . . You said, 'Listen now, and I will speak; I will question you, and you shall answer me'" (Job 42:2, 4 NIV). After that prayer God's plan for Job was revealed.

Even at her young age, Ella was ahead of Job in understanding that faith and trust precede revelation of the life job description. After this, "he makes everything work out according to his plan" (Ephesians 1:11).

Trusting ears alert
"This is the way, walk in it"
Looking back, it's clear

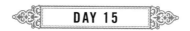

DAY 15

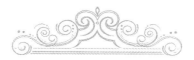

SINGING IN THE PAIN

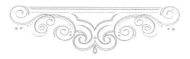

But as for me, I will sing about your power . . . For you have been my refuge, a place of safety when I am in distress.

—PSALM 59:16

BATH time with grandchildren is usually a happy time. My friend Gretchen says it's her favorite time of the day. Seeing the perfect little bodies covered with soap suds while chatting about the day's events and hearing the delighted squeals of little voices as they splash are a ritual she has used to bond close ties with her grandchildren.

Bath time with Ella is not so pleasurable. With her tiny body covered in open wounds and bandages that won't come off without causing more pain, even the thought of bathing causes her to burst into heart wrenching cries and begging for her mother not to make her get into the water. Infused with either bleach or special salt to fight possible infection, the water launches an agonizing assault on her already beleaguered skin.

But regular bath and bandage changes with application of special ointments and nonsticking bandages is currently the only treatment to protect the skin of a child with EB from infection and trauma. It is a necessary evil. Every child with EB hates bath time. Every parent or caregiver dreads the process.

For the first four years of her life, Ron and I couldn't bear to hear Ella's cries when we were visiting on bath day. The minute she sensed that her mother was getting things ready for the bath, she would begin to whimper. Blue eyes filled with tears and lips quivered. Katie switched to another place in her mind and detached from the hurt she must inflict. I left the house or locked myself in the basement where I couldn't hear.

It was also during bath and bandage change that Ella would question her mother about her disease. "Why doesn't God give me new skin?" she asked. "I pray every day for new skin. Mom, would you please ask God to give me new skin? I'm just a little girl. You're a grown up. He'll listen to you."

Baths are painful for Ella because of the irritation to her wounds. They are painful for Katie because there seems to be no way to comfort her daughter either physically or emotionally. Bath time is painful.

On a visit when Ella was five years old, as I stood at the bottom of the stairs listening and deciding if I should go out the door or wait inside, I heard something that made my heart both break and swell with gratitude. Ella was crying, but through her distress, she was singing praise songs to the Lord. She poured out her little heart in song to the only One she knew really understood what she was going through. Her sweet voice rang with longing, sincerity, and hope. She sang her way through the pain.

Most of us have found the solace that music provides during times of distress. In the days following the 9/11 attacks, I played praise music to quiet and calm my troubled soul. The last hours I spent with my mother in the hospital before she died, I played a tape of her favorite hymns and sang as we held hands—comforted as we said goodbye. Singing to our Lord is perhaps the purest form of worship. The words and the rhythm seem to be a conduit for emotional expression like nothing else. When words alone are not enough, we should sing.

Noise of heartbreaking
Transforms into melody
When song transposes

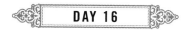

DAY 16

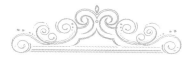

FINDING THE GOOD

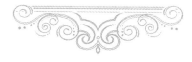

*If you plan to do evil, you will be lost; if you plan to do good,
you will receive unfailing love and faithfulness.*

—PROVERBS 14:22

FOUR sixth-grade girls sat around my kitchen table to plan a retirement party for their beloved teacher, Mrs. Hughes. The air was electric with excitement and great ideas. But there was one girl who couldn't seem to find the good in any part of the planning. Her comment to every suggestion was, "The trouble with that is . . ." and she would proceed to focus on every conceivable calamity that might befall whatever plans were being made.

How sad that one so young had already been programed to shut down good possibilities by listening with such a negative filter. Little by little, I saw the joy and energy in the other girls silenced. Excitement turned to frustration and self-doubt, then to defeat until they could no longer see the good in their ideas and almost decided to scuttle the whole idea of a party.

Suddenly, one girl slammed her hand on the table and said, "We're going to have a party for Mrs. Hughes, and it's going to be a really *good* party because she is a really *good* teacher and she needs a *good* party." And it happened just that way, and a good time was had by all. Thankfully, one girl saw the good.

Ella is one of those people who sees the good in everything. When you ask her how her day went, how school was, or how the trip to the doctor's office was, her answer is always the same: "Good." Her answer is sincere. In spite of pain and disability, having to sit and watch her friends play instead of participating, living a life of discomfort and exclusion that few can imagine, Ella always proclaims, "It's good."

Every year her parents take her to Cincinnati Children's Hospital EB Clinic for a thorough check up. For two or three days, she is ushered from one room to the next and examined by no fewer than a dozen doctors. Every inch of her delicate body is peered at and probed over. It isn't pleasant. How could it be? But at the end of the grueling schedule of exams and procedures as she was walking out of the hospital with her parents, she volunteered, "This hospital is really a fun place. All the doctors are so nice." When there were dozens of uncomfortable, painful invasions on her little body, Ella chose to exchange those memories for the smiling faces, soft voices, and tender touches of her caregivers.

Hospital visits and regular surgical procedures are a necessary part of Ella's life, but they are viewed by her friends as frightening. They fear for Ella. In her typical spirit of kindness and looking for the good, Ella told her mother before a trip to the hospital that she didn't tell her friends she would be absent from school because of a surgical procedure. Instead, she told them she was going to the dentist because she "didn't want them to be sad."

It's amazing that at her young age she has set her course on good and concern for others more than her own needs. In making this choice, she is fostering a heart of gratitude and strengthening herself for the time when finding the good in her situation will likely be more difficult.

Matthew 6:22 makes clear the benefit of looking for the good. "Your eye is like a lamp that provides light for your body. When your eye is healthy, your whole body is filled with light." Opening our eyes to focus on the good is sacrificial because we offer up self-pity and thank God for the ultimate outcome we know awaits.

Each time Ella says, "It's good" (and we know in our hearts it isn't), she is training her eyes to see the good and proclaiming her faith in God who makes all things right. With this attitude, she passes a bit of that good light along to others. She is training her eyes to see the good.

Sensing good in pain
Shedding a bit of light
Pain lessens and faith grows

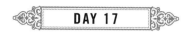

DAY 17

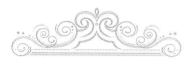

BEING BEN

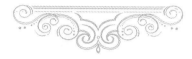

But ye are a chosen generation, a royal priesthood, an holy nation, a peculiar people; that ye should shew forth the praises of him who hath called you out of darkness into his marvelous light.

—1 Peter 2:9 KJV

C ARS *for sale 10 cents. Put money in bag.* The sign was duct taped to the fence post along with a ziplock bag. Customers were on the honor system to pay for each matchbox car they selected from the neatly arranged display on the sidewalk. On the day he opened his used car lot, Ben had decided it was time, at age eight, to start his own business. "I have too many cars, and other kids might not have so many and would appreciate a good deal." Ben has the mind of a financier and the heart of a philanthropist. He believes, "*Anything* is possible if you have faith" (Mark 9:23 TLB).

Included in a long list of passions are Ben's love of all cars, toy or real. Ask him about Ferraris and he can give a lengthy explanation of why one model is superior to another. One Saturday, Papa took his two grandsons on a trip to the local import dealership where Ben amazed the salesmen with his knowledge of their products. This young man is an expert in all things mechanical. Instead of reading typical children's literature, he pours over operating manuals and likes to discuss scientific processes and computers. Because I have known this boy's father and grandparents for several decades, I can verify that insatiable curiosity and zeal for life are in his DNA.

At first, Ben's parents simply thought him to be a very precocious toddler. But when his extraordinary intelligence and exuberant spirit was accompanied by troubling, unusual behaviors, an evaluation revealed a diagnosis of pervasive developmental disorder—not otherwise specified (PDD-NOS). Gradually the diagnosis became more evident in Ben's repetitive play skills and unusual sensitivity to sensory information, such as loud noises and lights. As he got older, his personality development was atypical. A tendency to impose social interactions on others brought a challenge to making friends. Being Ben wasn't easy. Change in routine or environment was difficult. When his family came back to his beloved Denver after a short move to Arizona, he sighed with relief, "Now all my dreams have come true."

While some children with PDD-NOS have communication and social aversions, Ben does not. In fact, he never meets a stranger, can engage conversation with anyone on a wide range of topics, and doesn't hold back in showing affection. So, what's the problem? The problem is that he has difficulty differentiating socially acceptable behaviors. The filter used to behave and communicate along social norms is different with Ben. He's a free spirit who says and does what he wants, and he runs wherever he goes. The regiment of a classroom is often difficult for him to navigate. He becomes quickly impatient and doesn't always know when or how to control the outpouring of creative observations and questions that pop into his head. Being Ben means navigating outside the umbrella of normal.

In this day, politically correct vocabulary vets most labels that suggest that a person is different from the norm. Social implication is that being "different" is not desirable. But God says several times in Scripture that those who are different have the most cherished place in His heart. In referring to the Children of Israel, His chosen people, He said, "Now therefore, if ye will obey my voice indeed, and keep my covenant, then ye shall be a peculiar treasure unto me above all people" (Exodus 19:5 KJV). Another translation of that scripture says they are "out of all nations . . . my treasured possession" (NIV). Evidently God looks with special affection on those who behave outside the norms of this world.

Ben loves, learns, and laughs with his whole heart. He read Jack London's *Call of the Wild* then insisted that the family move to Canada and start a preserve to protect wolves. After reading an article about cryogenics, he announced that he would become an expert in this field so that all the people who suffered from incurable diseases could be frozen until a cure was found. Where his tender heart sees a need, Ben looks for a solution.

The truth is, Ben's condition is not life-threatening, but it can be life altering for those who see his differences through a new lens. The behaviors that others label as disruptive and off-putting are in fact extensions of the characteristics we should nurture in any child: friendliness, confidence, exuberant energy, thoughtfulness, intelligence . . . and yes, persistent questioning, passions, and concerns. These come from a heart eager to love and learn. These traits are what it takes to be Ben.

Ben has a way of asking the big questions. At age five he paused in the middle of breakfast and asked, "Mom, what does it mean to exist?" If I were his mom, I would probably have rolled my eyes and said, "If I could answer that question I would be famous." Yet there is an answer to Ben's question and it is found in Titus 2:13–14 (KJV): existing is "looking for that blessed hope, and the glorious appearing of the great God and our Savior Jesus Christ; who gave himself for us, that he might redeem us from all iniquity, and purify unto himself a peculiar people, zealous of good works." God's definition of existing is to be different.

Want to be perfect?
Start outside the norm
Eager to do good

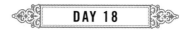

DAY 18

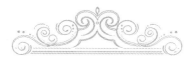

BECOMING A PRINCESS

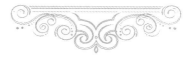

May he grant your heart's desires and make all your plans succeed.

—Psalm 20:4

LIKE most little girls, Ella went through a phase of princess obsession. She dreamed of castles, tiaras, and dancing in a beautiful dress at a palace ball. She wanted to be a Princess, and expected to have her wish granted. It happened in more splendid ways than she could have imagined.

Her first royal encounter was with Belle, Ella's favorite princess. She was invited to a private meeting prior to a performance of "Beauty and the Beast" at The John F. Kennedy Center for Performing Arts in Washington, DC.

For months afterward, Ella told anyone who would listen about meeting "the *real* Belle." Ask her why she likes Belle so much and she'll respond, "Belle likes to read books and is smart, and she was kind to the Beast even though he was mean and scary looking." To know that someone like Belle was undeterred by the outward visage of the Beast (or a little girl who was scarred and wrapped in bandages) touched Ella's heart, and she was comforted to know that not everyone judges others negatively because they look different.

The next encounter was at the Magic Kingdom. Our entire family went to Disney World when all three of our grandchildren were four years old. Their reactions were exactly what we hoped they would be . . . pure awe and wonder! Sam and Nate reveled in cowboys and cars. Ella wore a real Cinderella dress and had a transformation at the Bibbidi-Bobbidi Boutique. For the rest of the day, she moved and talked like the princess she had become.

The sign outside the final stop of the day, near the Main Street entrance said, *Meet the princesses*. Even though it was the end of a long, memorable day, we couldn't pass that up. As the rest of the family saved a curbside spot to view the grand finale electric parade, Ella, Katie, and I accepted the opportunity to be presented at court.

We made our way down the plush carpet of the elegant corridor where Ella had personal conversations with Cinderella, Sleeping Beauty, and Belle. She was breathless with delight. As we prepared to exit, the door guard asked if we could wait for just a moment until the other visitors exited. Not knowing what to expect, we moved to a corner to wait.

The Grand Hall emptied and the doors at either end of the hall were closed. The trio of princesses came to where Ella stood. Smiling with outstretched hands, they asked if they could spend some special time alone with her.

The royal trio led her to the center of the palace ballroom where Ella was initiated into a special sisterhood of real princesses. Their focus was totally on our girl as they chatted, compared ball gowns, sang and danced in an enchanted circle. Cinderella was particularly attentive, noting that they shared the same name and wore matching white, elbow length evening gloves . . . one of satin, the other of gauze. Katie and I tried to focus our cameras through tears as the Magic Kingdom lived up to its name.

Ella's desire to be a real princess was granted not just once, but twice. She dreamed big and got big results. Our own expectations are often mediocre and our dreams small. Perhaps we don't believe we have a right to big desires. Maybe we haven't yet learned to trust God to make dreams come true. Or it could be that we're scared to be a part of something that can only be explained as a work of God. Possibilities can seem to be out of our reach, but the King of Glory sees us as worthy of grand designs and longs for us to ask and believe.

Princess or pauper
When God's allowed to be God
Royalty is in us all

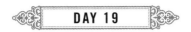

DAY 19

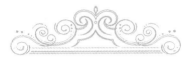

DR. MOM

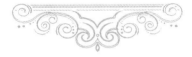

So let us come boldly to the throne of our gracious God.
There we will receive his mercy, and we will find grace to help us
when we need it most.

—Hebrews 4:16

LIKE most young girls, my daughter Katie spent a lot of time talking and dreaming about what she wanted to be when she grew up. After breaking her arm on the jungle gym at school, she wanted to be a bone doctor. In the 1980s, when big hair was the rage, she wanted to be a hairdresser. After going to her first Amy Grant concert, she wanted to be a Christian pop singer. High school speech competition inspired her to be the next great TV talk show hostess. The aspiration that lasted longest was to be a doctor . . . until her high school guidance counselor explained how many extra years of schooling it required.

I always felt Katie would have been a great doctor. She was interested in all things medical, even winning a blue ribbon for her science fair project on how to set a broken bone. Going fishing with her dad, she begged to do the gutting. When he brought deer or antelope home from a hunt, Katie stood at his side to observe the butchering process. She was never squeamish around blood and didn't turn pale or gag at cuts or scraped knees. She had the mind, heart, and fortitude to make a good doctor. All that kept her from pursuing that profession was the thought of those many years of school. Not for her.

Instead, Katie had a career in politics and governmental affairs until her daughter was born. Being such a rare disease, even in a large population area like Washington, DC, there was no one with experience treating EB. The best resources for Ella's care were the parents of other EB children. Even with such support, the disease reacts differently on each child, and the care must be customized through a lot of trial and error. Daily care is best managed by the family, and mom is usually the one to shoulder most of the responsibility.

Because the bath and bandage process is long, tedious, and painful for the child, even the most willing and capable mom can be overwhelmed and discouraged by the responsibility. Having your child scream and beg you to stop touching them goes against everything we are taught that mothering should be. But the EB mom silences the screams in her mind in order to perform the ritual that protects her child from additional skin trauma and life-threatening infection.

People often try to commend Katie and Joe for their extraordinary patience and care of Ella. Like most parents of children with special needs, they don't want to hear that they are exceptional. "I'm a mom. I just do what any mom would do," she says. She does, however, give credit to the extra measure of confidence the Lord has provided for her caregiver role. Hebrews 13:5–6 promises her "I will never fail you. I will never abandon you. So we can say with confidence, the LORD is my helper, so I will have no fear."

At the conclusion of a particularly difficult bath and bandage session, Katie examined a wound on Ella's chest that wouldn't heal despite weeks of treatment. As she often does, Katie talked to herself and to Ella about what the next step should be.

Ella's brilliant blue eyes looked directly into her mother's brilliant blues and she said, "Mom you are a really good doctor. But you aren't a *real* doctor. You're a doctor because I made you one."

Life sometimes sets us on an unexpected path and assigns a task we don't feel capable of handling. We feel scared and insecure, but God's promise is to be our helper and give us the confidence needed to persevere. Mary watched helplessly as her son Jesus suffered on the Cross. Even as her mother's heart broke, she looked into His eyes with determined love and understanding. From His birth, she kept her awareness of His life mission a secret in her heart. As best she could, she prepared Him to accept His destiny, and when the time came, she stood quietly in the shadows where He could sense her presence. She suffered with Him but stayed outwardly strong. She did what mothers do.

Take the wheel, He says
Unmapped roads are my domain
Steer the way I point

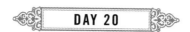

DAY 20

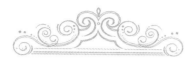

THIS LITTLE LIGHT OF MINE

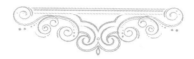

You are the light of the world . . . let your light shine before others,
that they may see your good deeds and glorify your Father
in heaven.

—MATTHEW 5:14–16 NIV

WORSHIP services at First Baptist Church, Alexandria, Virginia, are always uplifting, but Easter Sunday 2014 was especially so. Each moment of the service was fine-tuned to celebrate the Resurrection and life of Christ.

On this Easter Sunday, Ella's four-month-old brother A. J. (aka Abraham Joseph) was dedicated to the Lord with all the grandparents sitting in the center section on the second pew; close enough to reach out and touch the first chair violinist in the orchestra. After the dedication, A. J. and his family came down to join the grands. Ella sat in the middle of her extended family, beaming throughout the service. She sang each song with sincere gusto and listened attentively to the sermon and Scriptures. Ella loves to go to church, and she loves to sing.

When the service was over, many rushed to congratulate Katie and Joe on their new son. The grandparents stood proudly to the side, and Ella sat quietly watching. A woman walked from the orchestra carrying her violin. She paused and gazed at Ella with a compassionate smile on her face. I thought, "Please don't spoil this by asking what's wrong with the poor little girl." I held my breath until I heard her say to Katie, "You have the most beautiful daughter. I watched her through the entire service. The light of the Lord shines through her."

This violinist was new to the church and didn't know Ella or her story. She wasn't interested in her details but only wanted to say that she had been blessed by being in her light.

At Vacation Bible School, Ella memorized 1 Peter 3:15 (NIV): "But in your hearts revere Christ as Lord. Always be prepared to give an answer to everyone who asks you to give the reason for the hope that you have." The Scripture is another way of reminding us to shine our light. Whenever we are told that another sees our light, it is an affirmation that we are plugged in to the right power source.

Light vies with darkness
Illumination triumphs!
Power source revealed

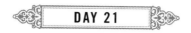

DAY 21

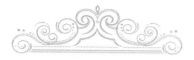

A FISH THAT WIGGLES

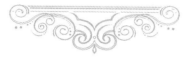

The thief comes only to steal and kill and destroy; I have come that they may have life, and have it to the full.

—JOHN 10:10 NIV

TAKING your grandchild fishing is part of being a grandfather. When my husband Ron talked to Ella as she lay in the incubator in the Neonatal Intensive Care Unit at National Children's Hospital, he told her to fight to get better so that one day he could take her fishing when she came to see us in Wyoming. At the time, fishing together was the very best thing he could wish for his first grandchild.

Four years later, we prepared for that first Wyoming fishing experience by buying the perfect pink fishing gear, complete with little pink plastic fish that could be caught with a magnet on the end of the line. We imagined our granddaughter casting, hooking, and reeling in the plastic fish. Just as we hoped, she was delighted with the pink rod and reel covered with princess decals. But after only one catch of a plastic fish, she looked at PawPaw and said, "This isn't a real fish. I want to catch a fish that wiggles." No counterfeit fishes for her!

Only a couple of days after her birth, Joe and Katie received an email from a woman in another town who they had never met. The message said simply that she was praying for Ella and that the Lord had put John 10:10 on her heart to share as a promise of hope for her life. Joe read the Scripture and immediately claimed it as his daughter's life verse: "The thief comes only to steal and kill and destroy; but I have come that they may have life, and have it to the full" (NIV).

As they claimed this promise for their daughter, Joe and Katie made a covenant with God to do everything possible to assure each day of Ella's life was meaningful and lived to the full. They would stand guard to prevent EB from stealing their hope and joy, killing their dreams for their child, or destroying life's abundant possibilities.

When a child is stricken by a sickness of monumental proportions, there is a tendency to isolate, limit interaction with the public, and erect an impenetrable wall of defense in an attempt to hold the ravages of the disease at bay. No one can fault parents for doing everything possible to keep their child safe, but in overly protecting from the bad it is possible to deprive them of the good. As a child is isolated from the bittersweet challenges of living this life, the thief can creep in to steal a bit of their confidence and curiosity, numbing them in some ways. Allowing experiences from as many spectrums as possible results in an abundant life that is authentic—not an imitation.

On a beautiful Wyoming August day, on the banks of Yesness Pond in Casper, Ella cast her fishing line into the water for the very first time, and stood patiently waiting for a tug on the hook. When it happened, PawPaw helped her to reel in her first fish. It was real and it wiggled!

See, do, taste and feel
Rich and satisfying life
The robber gets robbed

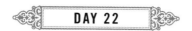

DAY 22

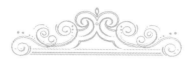

SWIMMING WITH BENJAMIN

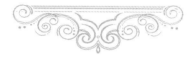

Even if my father and mother abandon me,
the LORD will hold me close.

—PSALM 27:10

ALEXANDER was helping his four-year-old brother Benjamin Noah learn to zip his coat. One-year-old Amelia was screaming because of a wet diaper, and three year old Isabelle was throwing a tantrum because the bows in her hair didn't match her dress. A typical morning, the O'Connell house was filled with loud, frantic activity. Megan and Ray reveled in the chaos!

Megan was born to be a mom. I've known her since she was two years old, when she would play for hours with her dolls. She had selected names for her future family before she was ten years old. But several years into her marriage with Ray, after hours of doctor consultations, prayer, and mourning the loss of the birth experience, the reality of infertility became painfully clear. The O'Connells fully embraced the option to fill their home with children through adoption.

First came Alexander (named for our family after the birth of Ella). An absolute joy of a boy, he announced at age three, "This house needs some more kids for me to play with." He got his wish a few years later when a call came from the local foster-to-adopt office. They had the baby girl Megan longed for. Only one day old, she was theirs with the stipulation that her 16 month old sister and two year old brother could come, too. Wow! Talk about answered prayer.

Megan and Ray opened their arms extra wide, traded their sports car for a minivan, and breathed deeply as they doubled the size of their family within 24 hours. They followed the promise expressed in Hebrews 2:13, "'I will put my trust in him,' that is, 'I and the children God has given me.'" Taking on a family of four small children required a lot of trust, along with patience, discipline, and a daily survival strategy.

Bath time for Benjamin was an unexpected battlefield. Unlike most children, Benjamin reacted violently to the sight of water filling the tub. He screamed, he ran, he fought, he cried with terror to the point of nearly passing out. He was inconsolably traumatized by water. Toys, calm talk, singing, bribery . . . nothing could soothe his bath time hysterics. After several weeks, Megan learned that this little boy's fear of water was well founded. He was a victim of child maltreatment, and had reasons not to trust bath water nor the one giving the bath.

Megan and Ray are not only calm, patient parents, they are also incredibly creative. They explored every avenue to help their son overcome his fear of water, including consulting a child behavior therapist for methods of relearning trust, safety, and self-soothing techniques. Finally, Megan learned of a program called "One Small Wish." She went to them with her dilemma and soon after received word that a series of swimming lessons had been arranged by an anonymous donor. It seemed like a good idea, but Megan couldn't help but wonder if her little boy was ready for a really large pool of water. During the first session, she and Alexander sat very close to the pool and big brother held Benjamin's hand as he slipped into the water.

As it turned out, water, the very source of Benjamin's terror and trauma, became the balm for healing that put him on the path to a healthy, happy life in his new family. With assistance from a trained, compassionate teacher, he learned to float, blow bubbles, and attempt to swim with joy. Benjamin's entire demeanor began to change. He smiled and splashed his water demon into submission! He went into the water a terrified child, but he came out a conqueror. Bath time is no longer a traumatic experience but a fun adventure that he looks forward to.

This passage from Revelation 7 seems to have been written to describe this one small boy: "For the Lamb on the throne will be their Shepherd. He will lead them to springs of life-giving water. And God will wipe every tear from their eyes" (v. 17).

The devastating effects of child maltreatment are deep and pervasive. The damage is seldom overcome with something as simple as swimming lessons. But we have to begin somewhere to save a generation of discarded children. Our response to these, the weakest, and sometimes invisible in our communities, should be a mirror of the character of Jesus in Mark 10:26–27, "'Then who in the world can be saved?' they [the disciples] asked. Jesus looked at them intently and said, 'Humanly speaking, it is impossible. But not with God. Everything is possible with God.'" Jesus invited the little children to come to him.

Some of us are afraid of water or of the unknowns lurking below its surface. When called by God to rescue a child or complete any heavenly assignment, we do well to dive in.

Afraid of water?
Float in the teacher's strong arms
The deep end beckons

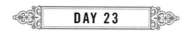

DAY 23

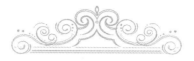

TOUCHING WORDS

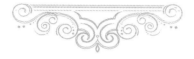

Wise words satisfy like a good meal;
the right words bring satisfaction.

—PROVERBS 18:20

SKIN is the body's largest organ; our first line of defense against the elements and infection. But apart from bemoaning my freckles as a teenager, and lathering my wrinkled face with lotion as an aging woman, I never gave it much thought until our granddaughter was born. Then my attitude toward skin and life changed forever.

Our precious baby girl was born with a very rare genetic skin disorder called epidermolysis bullosa . . . EB. Out of every 20,000 babies born, only one will have EB. Our Ella was that one. Her skin is fragile, like a butterfly's wings. Even the slightest friction produces painful blisters or agonizing open wounds that cover up to 75 percent of her tiny body. She has never been able to be touched, kissed, cuddled, or rocked to a lullaby without danger of her skin blistering or tearing. The protective function of her skin is impeded by the absence of collagen VII; result of the unfortunate collaboration of recessive genes from both her parents.

When she was born, we were told that EB is a condition for which there is currently no cure and that most EB children do not live to adulthood. The best treatment is bandages and ointments to protect from injury and infection.

We were told to tell Ella goodbye . . . that she wouldn't live.

I sat beside the incubator as she lay on a piece of lamb's wool. She was alone, isolated, and deprived of the thing I knew she needed to survive: human touch. That vital connection needed to be made, but how? Suddenly, I recalled a childhood memory. I was in tears because of a throbbing ear infection. My Nanny Wance crawled into bed beside me on the soft feather bed and began to tell me stories of her childhood escapades.

Soothed by her words, I fell asleep. I realized I could touch Ella with my words, my voice, with my breath, with my singing and with my softly uttered prayers.

Placing my cheek against the cold glass of the incubator, I whispered to Ella that she was strong—that she was loved—that she would live! I told her stories and read to her from the Bible of the healing miracles of our Heavenly Father, and I prayed for Him to send His angels to touch and hold her in my place. I told her about the world outside her incubator walls, and I told her that God had a very special plan for her life!

Reminded that "the words of the godly save lives" (Proverbs 12:6) and "the words of the wise bring healing" (v. 18) and following the example of Jesus who embraced the multitudes with stories, I talked, sang, read, prayed, and I touched that tiny girl with my words.

Words of caring, encouragement, and hope can be the stepping stones upon which we cross over the turbulent streams that run through life. There are times when the Lord impresses us to speak such words but we quench that urging and talk ourselves out of uncommon boldness. Caring words shared with daring can touch and heal even the most cynical and hardened heart.

Touch of skin ignites
Pleasure, pain, protection
Touch of words surpasses

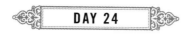

DAY 24

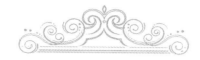

HEARING VOICE

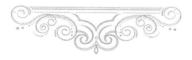

He calls His own sheep by name . . . they follow him because they know his voice.

—JOHN 10:3–4

E VERYONE called her Big Mama . . . grandchildren, in-laws, everyone in her small Texas community, and even grown men. The name suited her perfectly. Her laugh, her voice, her opinions, her jewelry, and her hair were all *big*. Wherever she went, she made a *big* impression. She was the first person I called whenever anything good or bad happened in my life. I never had to say, "This is Gale," and she never said, "This is Mama." We knew each other's voices. Her delight in my simple news made me feel valued. In the beginning, long distance calls were expensive so she kept an egg timer by the phone. Whatever needed to be said had to be said in three minutes or less. We learned to talk fast.

In her final years, with unlimited long distance rates, my day began with coffee, a crossword puzzle, and calls to Mama. She did most of the talking while I listened. She always ended the unhurried discourse by telling me how much she looked forward to the daily calls and how they caused the thousand miles between us to shrink.

Big Mama was a child of the Great Depression, raised as a sharecropper's daughter in a small house at the end of a long muddy lane. To her, the telephone was a magical instrument. At one point, there were 13 telephones in her house! Her final acts of friendship and ministry were with her beloved telephone in one hand and a list of those needing a call in the other. Always her conversations were "full of grace, seasoned with salt" (Colossians 4:6 NIV). No one will ever be as grateful for the wonders of a telephone as my mother.

Now my daily phone calls are with my granddaughter. She's the one I call to share news of the new bunnies in the back yard, or the recipe for a new fancy dessert. I don't have to say,

"This is Gigi." When she hears my voice, she's ready to sit and listen. In similar fashion, I'm the one she calls to tell how many dollars are in her treasure box, relate new antics by her baby brother, and brag of how she pulled some tricks on Dad in a recent game of chess. I end each call by telling her how much I look forward to the daily calls and that they make her seem to be not so far away.

I'm glad that Ella and I don't text or tweet. We talk. We sit at an imaginary table and share a feast of words served on the silver platter of vocal melody. The human voice adds a dimension to a message that can never be replicated with finger taps on a keyboard. The lilt and laughter in Ella's voice travels straight down the aural canal into my heart and makes me happy.

Amid the noise of daily activity, keep an ear turned toward heaven to hear the voice of the Lord. While He does use Scripture text, He leaves tweeting to the birds and speaks to us directly.

Both blessing and curse
Technology needs boundaries
Old ways can be best

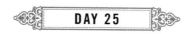
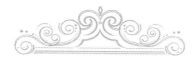

DOUBLE VISION

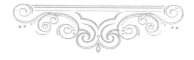

Let all bitterness . . . be put away from you.

—Ephesians 4:31 KJV

WALKING at my neighborhood mall not long after Ella was born, I paused to look in the window of a dance studio where a dozen little girls dressed as ballerinas in pink tutus were bouncing across the floor like sugarplum fairies. They were so beautiful, healthy, and perfect. Jealousy gripped my heart and I couldn't look at them. I had to turn and walk away.

Although I'm embarrassed to admit it, I was jealous of healthy babies. I didn't want to hold, hug, or even see pictures of them. Friends would proudly display images of their robust, rosy-cheeked grandchildren, but I had to manufacture interest and an appreciative half smile.

Jealousy is an evil emotion that can sap us of the ability to joyfully embrace life. Jealousy tainted the familial bond between Cain and Abel, Jacob and Esau. Whenever we want something someone else has, a covetous wall can separate us. I had head knowledge of this. I knew it was wrong. I prayed for the Lord to erase the resentment from my heart and, as is so often the case, God answered my supplication with a double dose of conviction.

On February 3, 2008, just eight months after Ella's birth, our son and his wife brought twin boys into our lives. The first time I held Sam and Nate—one in each arm—the shroud of jealousy fell away, and I fell totally in love. God knew I needed a double dose of healing, and a double vision to see just how much He loves me. Knowing of His individualized love for me makes it almost impossible to be jealous of anyone or anything.

In the medical realm, double vision is a problem. Two images of the same thing can cause dizziness and imbalance. But spiritual double vision is precisely the way Christians should see things; our view and His. Corrected vision comes when we acknowledge our own myopic perspective and make a heavenly correction. Having double vision can free us from self-centeredness, intolerance, and jealousy. This kind of sight allows us to see all things more clearly and opens our hearts to fully appreciate the blessings our Lord wants to give us. Sam and Nate taught me this.

The lens is cloudy
Add another . . . heaven's eyes
Two views are better

30 DAYS OF HOPE

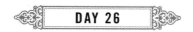

DAY 26

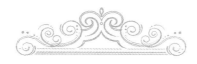

RUNNING WITH PURPOSE

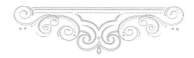

So I run with purpose in every step. I am not just shadowboxing.

—1 Corinthians 9:26

Our son Curby is a runner. In high school, college, and his younger bachelor days, he ran daily and scheduled long distance races monthly. Marriage, graduate school, and twin boys later, running was still in his heart but not on his schedule. Like the rest of us, he wanted to make a statement for his niece, Ella, and through a series of serendipitous events, found a group of EB family and friends who formed a team to run in the Cowtown Marathon where he lives in Fort Worth, Texas.

More than 20,000 runners would represent dozens of worthwhile causes, but Curby's team ran to raise awareness for EB and generate money through donations that would go toward EB research. Curby signed up to run the half marathon. No small statement for a man, age 42, who hadn't done any serious running for several years. Never one to do anything halfway, he went into full training mode. His goal was to finish the half marathon and not embarrass himself or disappoint his family who would be cheering at the finish line. He trained with purpose because he never does anything halfheartedly and because people would be watching him.

Curby and Gina mindfully teach their young sons to engage in meaningful activities that benefit others, and wanted to include Sam and Nate in running for the EB cause. Their sixth birthday came just weeks before the marathon, and with a little prompting from their parents, their birthday party invitation requested: No gifts. Donations for Dad's race to help fund research for EB would be appreciated.

The family had a cause to run for. Next, they needed a plan. Curby put together a page on their family blog and posted it to Facebook. Putting feet to the plan, he started each day a little earlier to have time to train . . . the more Curby ran, the more donations came in. Co-workers at Texas Christian University were recruited to run with the team, and friends from around the country donated money for the race.

The day of the big race finally arrived, and the experience was amazing. It was fun to see the EB running shirts in the crowd of 20,000 and to get to know the families. Some of the runners had an EB child in their family, while other people were friends. Some folks had heard about this disease through blogs or news stories and just wanted to be involved. The team goal was to raise $8,012.13 (because the EB child for whom the race was organized was born on August 12, 2013). The final tally was $9,600.00.

Ella's daddy comes from a family of athletes. His siblings organized fundraising runs in New Jersey and South Carolina. The humbling thing about going beyond yourself on behalf of others is that it's contagious, and you join with incredible people along the way to forge a common bond.

Most of us have an interest or talent that makes us come alive, and when we do it on behalf of others who can't, the reward of doing it is multiplied. Curby and the Murray clan use running. Even though each penny raised for EB research is appreciated, the real value of the races run by these aunts, uncles, cousins, and friends is that they demonstrate to Ella that she is not alone with her disease.

Telling a sick person that you care about them is one thing. Giving away your birthday or tying on sneakers and pounding the pavement as a physical statement of your support is quite another. That's real . . . not just shadowboxing.

Watching from the edge
Curious apathy
Smiles when purpose wins

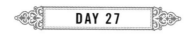
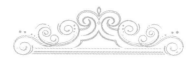

WHAT WERE WE TALKING ABOUT?

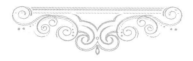

Two people are better off than one, for they can help each other succeed. If one person falls, the other can reach out and help. But someone who falls alone is in real trouble . . . three are even better, for a triple-braided cord is not easily broken.

—Ecclesiastes 4:9–12

OUR women in Casper, Wyoming, met in 1990 as actors in a community theater production of *Steel Magnolias*. After the production was over, their friendship continued and grew into a 20 year conversation that has touched on the widest array of topics, experiences, and emotions. Because the friendship seemed to encourage the strength and beauty in each of us to blossom, Gretchen, Vickie, Linda, and I began to refer to ourselves as the Wyoming Magnolias.

In the fall of 2007, a few months after Ella's birth, we four traveled from Wyoming to Natchitoches, Louisiana, for a girls' weekend getaway. We stayed in the very house where the movie *Steel Magnolias* was filmed. On that weekend trip, we were inspired to write and produce a stage play to use as a fundraiser for EB research. Ideas were jotted down on napkins and scraps of paper. Enthusiasm was palpable! Magnolia power infused four creative minds.

Over the next several years, the "Magnolias" met regularly to collaborate on a script that would come to be titled, *What Were We Talking About?* This seemed the perfect title for a play about the conversation that bounces between women who are good friends and love to talk. The result was a two-act play, based upon our personal stories of life altering challenge and triumph. The play celebrates the value of words, stories, and friendship while raising awareness about EB.

Without hesitation, each of the friends committed themselves to this project. Many hours of toil, sweat, laughter, and tears would be poured into this singular purpose. As Ella's grandmother, I pulled out all the stops. That's what grandmothers do. But my three friends sacrificed, agonized, and devoted themselves to this endeavor in a way that exemplifies the selfless goodness in the human spirit.

A simple, yet poignant line in the play is, "Things don't always turn out the way we plan." The visions of the good life we had in our twenties fade in our forties. Freakish accidents happen and change the course of a promising future. Some babies aren't born healthy, and deserving couples don't always give birth to the babies they yearn to hold. Yet, we continue to make plans while thinking that a strong woman can make things better.

What I experienced in the writing, producing, and performing of our play was spiritual direction that overrode our human plans, causing things to turn out better than we expected. Our plan was to have some fun while raising a few dollars for EB research. God's plan was bigger and better. After four years of extraordinary effort, uncounted hours of rehearsal and time donated by dozens of people, we premiered the play to full houses and standing ovations. The play has gone from Wyoming to New Jersey to Kentucky to Texas. Who can imagine the next venue? *What Were We Talking About?* has raised a lot of money for EB research and aid to EB families. It has educated many people about the disease, demonstrated tangible and emotional support to Ella's family, and taught four friends the power of a shared vision and allowing our dreams to be bigger than our practical expectations.

My favorite line from the play is, "Life isn't fair to any of us. It's how we handle the unfairness that defines us." The play reinforces what we all secretly yearn to believe: None of us needs to be alone in our suffering. We are all better when we link arms, forming a strong, unbreakable cord of shared hope and resilience to pull each other through the rough times.

Kindred hearts unite
To make a sacred statement
We are not alone

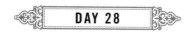

DAY 28

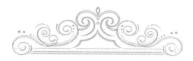

SHEDDING LAYERS

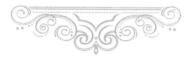

Forget the former things; do not dwell on the past.
See, I am doing a new thing!
Now it springs up; do you not perceive it?

—Isaiah 43:18–19 NIV

AFTER a premier in our hometown, my friends and I were invited to perform our play in Spring Lake, New Jersey, in October of 2013. This meant that rehearsals would be held during the fall school semester. Our director is a teacher, so the timing was not good. We needed help, and asked Cindy, a beautiful, creative woman, who agreed to step in as co-director. Inspired with sensitivity and heavenly insights, Cindy's involvement brought the message of our play to a whole new level.

There is a particular section titled, "Not the Woman I Used to Be." Here the characters speak of the changes that life's challenges have brought to our views of ourselves and others. For most of my life, I have known exactly who I am. When challenges came my way, I smoothly slipped into problem solver mode and moved forward. In most situations I was confident, optimistic, and resilient. With Ella's birth, that person ran for the hills. In her place stood a scared, confused woman who had no answers and no confidence to face an unexpected, unfamiliar adversary—I learned I have limits. I changed.

We thought the message of our play was: "Change makes you stronger." Cindy saw something very different, and led us to express transformation in a way we had not considered. She pointed out that the butterfly is the universal symbol for EB because the skin of a child with this disease is as fragile as a butterfly's wings. Even though their blistered and torn skin undergoes regeneration, it never completely heals. The result is skin that is weaker and more vulnerable . . . not stronger. Shedding the layers of damaged skin takes the child to new levels of vulnerability. Similarly, a butterfly goes through more than its share of traumatic metamorphosis, and when it finally reaches splendid maturity, its season of fragile beauty is much too short.

Cindy understood that a new creation is fragile . . . like a delicate butterfly. When a child with special needs comes into your life, it changes the lens through which you look at the world and it tests the limits of your own self-perception. Thinking it a sign of weakness, I had never been one to freely shed tears. But crying for Ella opened the floodgates and allowed me to experience the cleansing that comes from weeping. Because the days afforded to an ill child are often cut short, we learn to revel in small victories and joy-filled moments that catch us by surprise. Each day is a delicate treasure.

The four women in our play were directed to honestly acclaim that we were no longer the strong women we once thought we were as we unfurled the wings on a gigantic, breathtakingly beautiful butterfly at center stage. The physical display of how even painful change can result in beautiful transformation brought the audience to its feet!

Honestly shedding layers can put us into a fragile new place in the here and now. I find that I am more transparent, less concerned with presenting an impressive public image, and more open to talking about my own failed dreams, missteps and dark secrets. Freeing myself to tell my story made me hungry to hear the stories of others. Accounts of victory give me faith in humanity and reaffirm my view of God's right.

As we mature, shed layers, and adapt to life challenges, we become more vulnerable and aware of our own frailties and the need for others, especially the Divine Other, to help us through the transformation process. Accepting the cycle of change and jumping into the unknown to become new takes faith and courage.

Old friend in the mirror
Who's standing in your shadow?
One I want to know

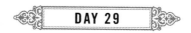

DAY 29

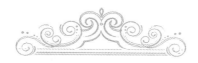

CHASING ADEN

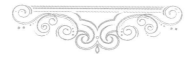

*Let us strip off every weight that slows us down...and let us run
with endurance the race God has set before us.*

—Hebrews 12:1

With his helmet strapped on tight, fingers clutching the handlebars, feet firmly planted on the pedals, five-year-old Aden was ready for his first ride on a two wheel pedal bike. After a gentle push, he went lickity-split down the deserted back street with Dad running behind yelling, "Look out for that trailer!" Aaron chased his son, caught up and grabbed him just as the bike was veering straight toward the obstacle in his path.

That's pretty much how it is with Aden as your son. Riding a bicycle, dancing with acrobatic abandon, wrestling with his sister, and jumping off furniture are all part of being this young boy. You might expect a few broken bones from any feisty risk-taker, but this little guy has had more than his share of fractures. Born with a rare genetic fragile bone condition called OI, even ordinary child's play can result in a trip to the emergency room, weeks in a cast, and painful immobility for Aden.

Osteogenesis imperfecta (OI) affects only six or seven out of 100,000 people worldwide. There are eight types of this condition. With Type 1, the bones get stronger as a child gets older, but with more severe types, disabling, painful, and life threatening issues ensue. Aden has Type III-IV, meaning he should not have expected to walk, much less ride a bike. He is no stranger to the emergency room and has had several breaks to his femur that kept him immobile for weeks at a time. Surprisingly, he seldom complains about the pain or being confined to his bed, using the time to strum his little guitar and make up songs.

Aden now has steel rods in both legs and was told he would most likely need to use a wheelchair. The wheelchair is stored in the basement . . . unused. Bottles of pain medication his mom was told would be needed are rarely opened. Chasing a full and happy life, this kid walks, runs, jumps, and defies all the doubters. Paul's words of encouragement to the Corinthians seem to fit Aden and his family: "We are pressed on every side by troubles, but we are not crushed. We are perplexed, but not driven to despair. We are hunted down, but never abandoned by God. We get knocked down, but we are not destroyed" (2 Corinthians 4:8–9).

Even though his condition has destined him to be smaller than most children his age, Aden has a personality and presence that make him a giant! When he walks into a room and flashes his infectious smile, others see a gregarious boy who makes friends with anyone willing to listen to his chatter or a song he has composed on his guitar.

Along with a big personality, Aden has a very big faith in God. He and his family are part of an amazing fellowship of support at College Heights Baptist Church in Casper, Wyoming. He first came into the community of believers when he was just six weeks old and has lived his life buffered by a soft circle of family and friends who have held him gently throughout his journey with OI. A mighty prayer warrior, every day he prays to Jesus, "Thanks that I didn't break a bone today. Help me not break a bone tomorrow." Hearing his earnest prayers has strengthened the faith of his parents and extended family. Chasing Aden means trying to keep up with him both physically and spiritually.

Nicole and Aaron look to Scripture for encouragement in raising their son. They stumble, are discouraged, lose hope, and then remember God's promises and pick themselves up for the next leg of the race. "The godly may trip seven times, but they will get up again" (Proverbs 24:16).

Is this so very different from the daily lives most of us lead? Parents chase after their children, shout out warnings, and grab them when they get too close to the precipice. We all chase after a full and happy life, but our pace is at times painfully slow because we are encumbered with the weight of sin and self-doubt. To run the race with endurance we must keep our eyes on Jesus. "For the LORD protects the bones of the righteous; not one of them is broken" (Psalm 34:20).

Aden is a happy, optimistic, gregarious child who brings sunshine everywhere he goes. Chasing him is a joyful privilege and those who run after him are exhilarated by the race.

> *Racing toward the goal*
> *Stripping earthly doubt and fear*
> *Weight transforms to wings*

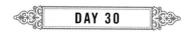

DAY 30

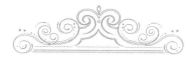

FRAGILE BUT FIERCE

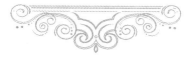

*God hath chosen the weak things of the world to confound the
things which are mighty.*

—1 CORINTHIANS 1:27 KJV

I'M NOT exactly sure when it happened, but there was a point during that first year after Ella's birth that my heart and my eyes were opened to see that EB children didn't have an exclusive claim on the trait of fragility. Friends and acquaintances would ask about her condition and follow my response with, "Let me tell you about *my* experience with a sick child." I discovered that our family was part of a very large group where each had a story to tell. Most were stories of how hope and faith triumphed over despair and how a child fought off the shackles of a disability or disease to live a happy, purposeful life.

Most of the stories came from people I knew well, yet I had never heard them speak of the fear and uncertainty that comes with having a child with an incurable condition. I had heard the story of a grandson who made the All Star soccer team in his state, but had not heard that he did it with prosthetic legs because he was born without those limbs. I had heard of a granddaughter's blue ribbons in equestrian competitions but not that she was autistic. Caleb, Ben, Schuyler, Benjamin, and Aden are children from families with which I have deep, long-standing personal connections. Through them, I have learned that every story has two sides and that we have a choice about which side becomes our story. A child's sickness can be the focal point of their story, or it can be a footnote.

My husband once asked me, "Suppose God answered our prayer for healing Ella from EB but there was one condition: EB had to be replaced with another disability and we were to pick what it was. Which infirmity would you choose?" That's when it dawned on me that we are all fragile. Ella has fragile skin that is out there for all to see. Others have less obvious weaknesses. We pass them in our daily walk without sensing their inner pain. Physical, mental, spiritual, emotional, and moral frailty permeate our world. Such shortfalls call us to treat each other with uncommon kindness.

Several years after Ella had her princess dreams fulfilled at the Magic Kingdom, the Murrays returned to the Hollywood Studios park at Disney World. Princess obsession had been replaced by the Force of Star Wars. She enrolled in jedi training school, fought Darth Vader, and won! Telling me of the experience, she said, "GiGi, if you ever go there, listen for the Star Wars music and go see Darth Vader. I think he will remember me because he said, 'This jedi is small, but she is powerful.'"

Gideon was among the least impressive of God's soldiers, but his weakness became strength in God's hands and he saved the Israelites from destruction by the Midianites. My sister-in-law, Kay, was a tiny, fragile lady whose body was broken by cancer, but her life and spirit soared above her weakness to be a mighty example of God's peace. Ella, Caleb, Ben, Schuyler, Benjamin, and Aden are warriors with weaknesses that God is using to display His love, grace, and power. Each is fragile, but their determination and courage are fierce.

The stories of our lives should likewise proclaim "He gives power to the weak and strength to the powerless" (Isaiah 40:29).

Weakness in us all
Fragile bodies, minds, & souls
Fire makes steel from clay

Also in the "Gifts of Hope" series...

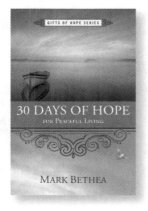

30 Days of Hope for
Peaceful Living
Mark Bethea
ISBN-13: 978-1-59669-437-8
N154115 · $9.99

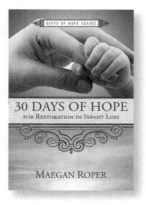

30 Days of Hope for
Restoration in Infant Loss
Maegan Roper
ISBN-13: 978-1-59669-438-5
N154116 · $9.99

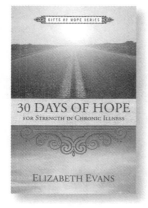

30 Days of Hope for
Strength in Chronic Illness
Elizabeth Evans
ISBN-13: 978-1-59669-465-1
N164105 · $9.99

Coming Fall 2016

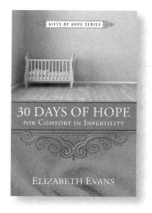

30 Days of Hope for
Comfort in Infertility

Elizabeth Evans

ISBN-13: 978-1-59669-464-4

N164104 · $9.99

(Available September 2016)

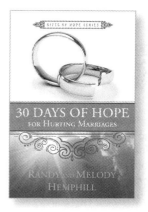

30 Days of Hope for
Hurting Marriages

Randy and Melody Hemphill

ISBN-13: 978-1-62591-507-8

N174106 · $9.99

(Available October 2016)

 For information, visit NewHopePublishers.com.

Please go to
NewHopePublishers.com
for more helpful information about
30 Days of Hope for Joy through a Child's Severe Illness.

If you've been blessed by this book,
we would like to hear your story.
The publisher and author welcome your comments and
suggestions at: newhopereader@wmu.org.